# A GUIDE TO HEMATOLOGY
## IN DOGS AND CATS

Suzanne
Tiemstra
# 686.8327

# A GUIDE TO HEMATOLOGY
## IN DOGS AND CATS

**Alan H. Rebar DVM, Ph.D., Diplomate, ACVP**
Purdue University
School of Veterinary Medicine
West Lafayette, Indiana

**Peter S. MacWilliams DVM, Ph.D., Diplomate, ACVP**
University of Wisconsin-Madison
School of Veterinary Medicine
Department of Pathobiological Sciences
Madison, Wisconsin

**Bernard F. Feldman DVM, Ph.D**
Virginia-Maryland Regional College of Veterinary Medicine
Department of Biomedical Sciences and Pathobiology
Blacksburg, Virginia

**Fred L. Metzger Jr., DVM, Diplomate, ABVP**
Metzger Animal Hospital
State College, Pennsylvania

**Roy V. H. Pollock DVM, Ph.D.**
Fort Hill Company
Montchanin, Delaware

**John Roche, M.S.**
Hematology Systems
IDEXX Laboratories
Westbrook, Maine

Teton NewMedia
*Innovative* Publishing
Jackson, Wyoming 83001
www.veterinarywire.com

Executive Editor: Carroll C. Cann
Development Editor: Susan L. Hunsberger
Editor: Cynthia J. Roantree
Design & Layout: Anita B. Sykes
Printer: Sun Litho

Teton NewMedia
P.O. Box 4833
4125 South Hwy 89, Ste. 1
Jackson, WY 83001
1-888-770-3165
www.veterinarywire.com
www.tetonnm.com

Cover Photo, not including blood cell photos: www.comstock.com

Chapter 11 is modified with permission from Ralston Purina Company; Hemogram Interpretation for Dogs and Cats, Ch 4; Alan H. Rebar, DVM; ©1998

QBC and VetAutoread are trademarks of Becton Dickinson and Company. All other product and company names and logos are trademarks of their respective holders.

The authors and publisher have made every effort to provide an accurate reference text. However, they shall not be held responsible for problems arising from errors or omissions, or from misunderstandings on the part of the reader.

PRINTED IN THE UNITED STATES OF AMERICA

ISBN # 1-893441-48-2


Print number 5 4 3

        Library of Congress Cataloging-in-Publication Data
IDEXX Laboratories guide to hematology / Alan H. Rabar ... [et al.].
    p. ; cm.
  Includes bibliographical references and index.
  ISBN 1-893441-48-2 (alk. paper)
    1. Veterinary hematology–Laboratory manuals. I. Title: Guide to hematology. II. Rebar, A. H. III. IDEXX Laboratories.
    [DNLM: 1. Hematologic Diseaeses–veterinary–Laboratory Manuals. 2. Laboratory Techniques and Procedures–veterinary–Laboratory Manuals. SF 769.5 I19 2001]
SF769.5 J34 2001
636.089′615–dc21

                                              2001027901

# Table Of Contents

# Acknowledgements

A book of this scope and magnitude would not be possible without the support and input of a number of key individuals. The authors gratefully acknowledge Ruth Ann Weiderhaft and Heather March for their role in facilitating communications among the authors and publishers and for keeping the authors "on task". Heather also played a significant role in producing the photomicrographs in the text. We also thank Dr. Karen Thomason, Dr. Bernard Feldman's wife and a James Herriott type of veterinary practitioner, for keeping us in touch with the realities of everyday veterinary practice. Finally we thank the outstanding team members of the Metzger Animal Clinic for their daily patience, commitment and dedication.

# Preface

This text is designed to assist the practicing small animal veterinarian in the interpretation of hematologic data. Emphasis is placed on both the quantitative (numeric) and qualitative (morphologic) evaluation of blood cells.

After a brief consideration of in-clinic approaches to hematology and available cell measurement methodologies (Chapters 2-3), the early chapters of the book (Chapters 4-10) systematically discuss the normal, abnormal, and artifactual findings for each cellular component of blood. The modified outline approach is intended to provide practitioners with quick and easy access to important information regarding a variety of hematologic abnormalities. However, the book is not intended as a complete treatise on hematology. For this purpose, readers are referred to excellent reference texts such as *Schalm's Veterinary Hematology* and John Harvey's *Atlas of Veterinary Hematology*.

The latter chapters of the book (Chapters 11-12) illustrate an integrated and systematic approach to hemogram interpretation. Case studies (Chapter 12) will hopefully allow practitioners to practice and develop their interpretive skills and confidence. In addition, these cases illustrate the scope of abnormal hemograms encountered. While hemogram interpretation can indeed be challenging, rewards to both the practitioner and patient can be profound.

# 1

# How To Use
# This Guide

This guide was developed as a practical hands-on resource for veterinarians and veterinary technicians in small animal practice.

We believe that hematology is one of the most useful, and most under-utilized, diagnostic tools in veterinary practice. The composition of the blood changes early in response to disease. Blood is readily obtained and, with modern instrumentation, is quickly and inexpensively evaluated. A complete hemogram provides a wealth of information about a patient's health or condition.

Our objective is to support the increased use of hematology in clinical practice by providing information in a concise, easy-to-find manner. We have chosen an outline format and kept the text to a minimum. The discussion of each cell type follows the same general outline:

Overview

Quantity
 Normal
 Decreased
 Increased

Morphology
 Normal appearance and variation
 Abnormalities
 Artifacts

Emphasis has been placed on clinical application. Detailed discussions of ultrastucture, physiologic, and biochemical pathways are covered in longer texts. Cell icons are used to facilitate locating the appropriate section, and both normal and abnormal morphology are profusely illustrated. Multiple Choice Questions and Case Studies are included to encourage self-evaluation and integration of principles.

# HOW TO USE THIS GUIDE

1. Keep it open in the office laboratory.

2. Use in-clinic hematology instruments or a commercial laboratory to obtain a complete blood count.

3. Evaluate the cell morphology on stained smears.

4. Refer to the sections on 'Interpreting the Hemogram" and to specific blood cell type(s).

5. Check the causes of quantitative disorders and the patterns of findings that suggest specific disease processes.

6. If you encounter abnormalities that you cannot characterize or that are beyond the scope of this book, consult a board certified veterinary clinical pathologist at a university or commercial laboratory.

7. Utilize hematology and this Guide consistently until it becomes a routine aspect of clinical care in your practice.

# LIMITATIONS OF THIS GUIDE

This guide is intended as a practical handbook for practitioners. As such, it does not cover all the known blood disorders of the dog and cat or contain detailed discussions of pathophyisiology. Excellent in-depth reference texts, such as *Schalm's Veterinary Hematology*, are available. No guide can substitute for advanced training and experience in rare or complex disorders. We strongly encourage consulting with specialists on difficult or unusual cases.

# 2

# Hematology
# In Practice

# INDICATIONS FOR HEMATOLOGY

The complete blood count (CBC) provides a broad overview of the general health status of the patient.

▶ Peripheral blood serves as a transport medium between the bone marrow and tissues.

▶ The CBC therefore provides a "snap-shot" of the hematopoietic system at a specific point in time.

Complete blood counts are recommended in the laboratory evaluation of every sick patient, every pre-anesthetic evaluation, every senior/geriatric profile, and as a recheck test for patients previously diagnosed with erythrocyte, leukocyte, or platelet abnormalities.

▶ Note that the definition of sick includes those patients with vague histories such as:
  – Not eating well
  – Unwilling to play
  – Has less energy

▶ Erythrocyte, leukocyte, and platelet abnormalities should be evaluated prior to anesthesia for several important reasons:
  – Anemic patients are more prone to tissue hypoxia, which increases the likelihood of anesthetic complications.
  – Polycythemia most commonly results from dehydration (relative polycythemia). Dehydration may cause hypotension and may result in anesthetic complications especially when coupled with blood loss and the vasodilitory effects of many anesthetic agents.
    ◆ Elevated total protein and concentrated urine specific gravity are other laboratory abnormalities associated with dehydration.
  – Leukocytosis may be associated with inflammation, stress, or excitement (physiologic leukocytosis).
  – Leukopenic and neutropenic patients may have difficulty in mounting an effective anti-inflammatory response postoperatively.
  – Thrombocytopenia is the most common bleeding disorder in veterinary medicine. Platelets must be evaluated in every pre-anesthetic test because the consequences of thrombocytopenia can be life threatening.

▶ Because it is an excellent screening tool which provides a wealth of information at relatively low cost, we recommend pre-anesthesia hematology and chemistry for all surgical candidates regardless of age.

► Geriatric patients, both healthy and ill, are also prime candidates for laboratory testing. Annual screening is recommended for healthy dogs and cats over the age of 7.

– Blood profiling provides important clues to underlying often unrecognized diseases and helps establish baseline data, nutritional, and vaccine recommendations.

♦ The minimum senior canine database includes the history (including behavior), physical exam, CBC, biochemical profile with electrolytes, and complete urinalysis.

♦ The minimum senior feline database includes the history (including behavior), physical exam, CBC, biochemical profile with electrolytes, complete urinalysis, and total T4.

– Aging is associated with an increased incidence of a variety of disease states which may be recognized first on the basis of abnormalities in the CBC, urinalysis, and/or chemistry profile. These include:

♦ Immune-mediated disorders

♦ Endocrinopathies such as diabetes mellitus, hyperadrenocorticism (Cushing's disease), thyroid dysfunction, and hyporadrenocorticism (Addisons' disease)

♦ Renal disease

♦ Hepatic disease

♦ Neoplasia

– Senior/geriatric laboratory profiling is both good medicine and good business.

♦ A recent AVMA study reported that 28.1% of U.S. dogs and 25.4% of U.S. cats were 8 years of age or older

# IN-CLINIC VERSUS OUTSIDE LABORATORY

Advantages of in-clinic hematology capability include faster patient management, better pre-anesthesia management, and the minimization of artifacts caused by delayed analysis.

► Improved patient management results from earlier diagnosis and treatment.

– Clinicians can use in-house laboratory results to determine the patient's health status (sick or well), create diagnostic and treatment plans, and provide written estimates for clients during the same office call.

► Client compliance increases when pre-anesthetic testing occurs in-house because the pre-anesthetic profile is performed the same day as anesthesia therefore minimizing client inconvenience.

► Pre-anesthetic testing should be performed immediately prior to anesthesia to properly evaluate patient status and adjust anesthetic regimes.

► Hematology samples should be analyzed as soon as possible to prevent artifacts created by exposure to anticoagulants and cell deterioration due to storage and shipment.
  – Blood films should be prepared within 30 minutes of collection to avoid morphologic artifacts.
  – Platelet counts should be performed as soon as possible after collection for optimal results.

Potential disadvantages of in-clinic hematology include slightly higher cost/sample, the potential for less complete quality control depending on the in-clinic technology, and limited expertise in microscopic assessment of blood films.

► Concerns regarding quality control can be minimized by:
  – Running in-house controls on a daily basis and charting results to ensure that there is no instrument drift in the results.
  – Frequently splitting samples and checking in-house results against those of a quality reference laboratory.
  – Joining a national quality control survey such as that provided by the American Society of Clinical Pathologists.

► As long as in-house quality control is maintained, the slightly higher costs of in-house hematology can be easily justified on the basis of better service to the patient.

# COMMUNICATING THE NEED FOR HEMATOLOGY

Most clients understand that human diseases are usually diagnosed through testing. Make clients aware that you don't want to guess.

► Clients understand that doctors should base treatment decisions on diagnosis, not speculation.

Use simple terms and explain that blood tests are required to rule out common diseases people are familiar with like anemia, infection, diabetes, and kidney disease.

► Many clients are familiar with the term "CBC" and "chemistry panel" through medically oriented television shows.

► Explain that these tests are like puzzle pieces which doctors use to narrow the list of potential diseases (differential diagnosis).

Remember that "normal" results are good news to the client and not money wasted.

- ▶ "Normal" laboratory results are common and have great value.
- ▶ Laboratory testing is used to help rule out diseases as well as to help identify them!

## COMMUNICATING THE RESULTS

Copy the laboratory results page to discuss your findings with clients.

- ▶ If results are abnormal, recommend treatment or additional diagnostics such as cytology, radiography, ultrasonography, endoscopy, etc.
- ▶ If results are normal, advise clients what diseases you have ruled out (ie, diabetes, anemia, infection, kidney disease).

Provide more information by copying an article on the diagnosed disease from a textbook or other reference source. This reinforces your diagnostic efforts and provides treatment and prognostic information for the client.

## THE ECONOMICS OF LABORATORY TESTING

Laboratory testing is an important profit center for veterinarians and should represent approximately 20% of average gross income according to the 2000 Veterinary Economics Best Practice Survey.

- ▶ The same survey reported $30 as the average charge for a CBC in the United States. Regional charges varied from a low of $21 in the South to $31 in the Northeast.
- ▶ Multiple surveys have shown that laboratory testing is relatively price insensitive when compared to regularly shopped items like vaccines, office calls, and flea and heartworm preventatives.

In-house testing is generally more expensive than outside laboratory testing. Consequently, veterinarians should charge a higher fee for tests performed in-house and justify the higher charges on the basis of faster, more customized service.

# 3

# Laboratory Methods in Hematology

# BLOOD COLLECTION

Proper blood collection or handling is critical; improper technique can result in inaccurate blood cell counts and morphologic artifacts.

▶ Sample quality is the major contributor to analytical errors.

Hematological assessment requires liquid blood.

▶ Blood should be drawn into vials or syringes that contain anticoagulant. EDTA is the anticoagulant of choice for most hematology (Figures 3-1 and 3-2).
  – Smears should be prepared as soon after collection as possible; prolonged exposure to EDTA produces artifacts in neutrophils and platelets.
  – Red cells show increased susceptibility to lysis after 24 hours in EDTA.

▶ Sodium citrate is recommended for platelet and coagulation studies.

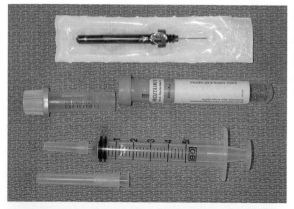

**Figure 3-1** Collection materials for hematological assessment include syringe, needles, and purple topped collection tubes that contain EDTA. Blood in tubes should be mixed by inversion rather than shaking.

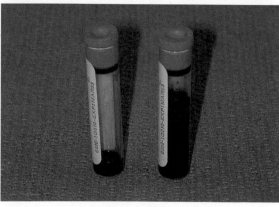

**Figure 3-2** EDTA tubes should be filled to their labeled capacity. Short filled tube (left) has an excessive amount of EDTA relative to the blood volume. Short filled tubes cause a false increase in total plasma protein content and a false decrease in PCV and RBC count. Shrinkage of RBCs causes a reduction in the MCV.

► Heparin should not be used to collect blood for canine and feline hemogram interpretation. It fails to prevent platelet aggregation and causes morphologic changes in white cells.

Self-drawing evacuated tubes (e.g., Vacutainer®, Becton Dickinson, Franklin Lakes, NJ or Monoject®, Kendall, Mansfield, MA) are preferred to syringes.

► They should be allowed to fill to capacity to achieve the appropriate blood/anticoagulant ratio (see Figure 3-2).

► Invert the vial several times after filling to ensure thorough mixing.

Rapid aspiration or transfer of blood with a syringe through a small gauge needle can cause cell lysis.

# HANDLING THE SAMPLE

Blood should be processed as soon as possible after collection.

► Blood films should be made immediately.

► If a delay is anticipated before processing further, the blood should be refrigerated.

► Excessive time at room temperature can cause autolysis.

► Platelet counts are most affected by delays in processing. Platelets have short life spans and tend to clump over time, even in the presence of anticoagulants. Platelet counts performed more than 4-6 hours after collection are suspect (See Figure 4-23).

Blood samples should be mixed again several times immediately before a portion is removed for testing; avoid prolonged mixing to prevent physical trauma to cells.

## Blood Films

Well prepared blood films are prerequisite to accurate assessment of the hemogram.

Use only new, clean slides.

Place a small drop of blood near the frosted end of one slide (Figure 3-3A).

► Place another slide at an angle of about 30 degrees to the first; draw back until it touches the drop of blood in the acute angle between the slides. (Figures 3-3B and 3-3C).

► After the blood has spread to within 2-3 mm of the edge, push the second slide quickly and smoothly across the full-length of the first (Figure 3-3C).

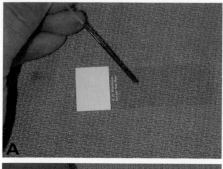
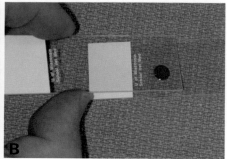
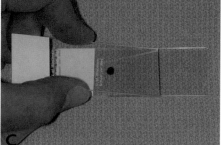

**Figure 3-3**

Preparation of a blood film. **A.** Small drop of blood is placed on a glass slide. **B.** and **C.** A second slide is used to spread the blood. Lowering the spreader slide produces a longer blood smear. Raising the spreader slide produces a shorter smear.

▶ A well formed smear has a flame shape.

▶ Prepare several slides from each patient.

An alternative method preferred by some hematologists is a variant of the coverslip method.

▶ Using a PCV tube, place a drop of blood slightly off center on a CLEANED (IMPORTANT) glass slide.

▶ Place a second cleaned glass slide on top and watch the spread of blood by capillary action between the two slides.

▶ Just as this stops, slip the upper slide off (DO NOT LIFT OFF!). This most often results in two thumbprint-sized perfect smears.

▶ The monolayered areas are the entire center of these smears with a thicker but small perimeter.

Air dry the smears quickly and store at room temperature until processed.

▶ Do not blot or wipe dry; this introduces scratches.

▶ Do not refrigerate; the condensation that forms on cold slides can lyse cells.

▶ Keep away from formalin.

▶ Do not fix until ready to stain, but keep covered; flies will consume blood on air dried smears.

# Staining

Romanowsky stains (Wright, Giemsa, and modified quick stains) afford the best overall morphologic assessment of the hemogram.

▶ These stains contain both an acid stain (usually eosin) and a basic stain (such as methylene blue).

▶ Structures rich in basic compounds, such as eosinophil granules, bind the acidic dye and are stained red. Acidic structures, such as DNA/RNA or basophil granules, are stained blue by the basic stain.

New methylene blue

▶ A supravital dye used for reticulocyte counts and to accentuate Heinz bodies.

▶ Mix a few drop blood with 1-2 times as much of 0.5% new methylene blue in physiologic saline, allow to stand a few minutes and use to make blood films.

# Common Artifacts/Issues

Stain precipitate

▶ Stain that is old or has been left open may deposit precipitate on the slide that can be mistaken for hemoparasites.

▶ Keep stain fresh and always covered when not in use. Periodically filter or replace to minimize precipitate.

Over- or under-staining

▶ It is often necessary to experiment with staining procedures to avoid over-staining or under-staining.

▶ In over-stained slides, all cells are deeply colored. The red cells appear to be more dense and more basophilic (blue) than normal. Over-staining can obscure important cell details (Figure 3-4).

▶ In under-stained slides, all cells are pale. Cellular details of the leukocytes are barely distinguishable and red cells are very faint. This should not be confused with hypochromia.

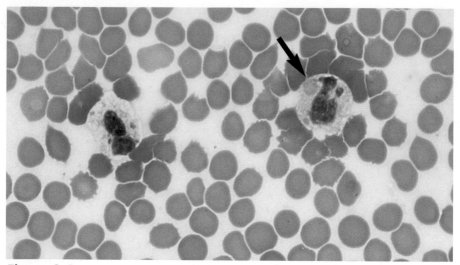

**Figure 3-4** Blood film that has been overstained with Wright Giemsa. The RBCs are a dark blue grey color that makes the identification of polychromasia impossible. The neutrophil on the right contains a canine distemper inclusion in the cytoplasm (arrow).

# SAMPLE EVALUATION
## Morphological Assessment

Microscopic examination of a blood smear is an essential part of any hematological evaluation, regardless of the method used to enumerate the cells.

▶ Blood cell counts alone are not sufficient to adequately evaluate the hemogram.

▶ The size, nature, and condition of cells and platelets provide information vital to characterize disease processes.

– Some diseases, for example, blood parasites and certain neoplasms, can be diagnosed directly from examination of the blood film.

A systematic approach to evaluation of the blood smear is essential to obtain accurate and complete results.

▶ A common error is to begin to identify and count the white cells immediately at high magnification, failing to observe the characteristics of the leukocytes, erythrocytes and platelets.

▶ Scan at low magnification (10-20X) for rouleaux formation and for RBC, WBC or platelet aggregation, which can cause erroneous cell counts in most automated counters.

– Estimate the total number of leukocytes (Figure 3-5) and develop

## Figure 3-5

Series of blood smears with increasing WBC counts. **A.** Blood film from a dog that is severely leukopenic and anemic. The density of RBCs and WBCs is markedly reduced. **B.** Blood film from a dog with normal WBC count. **C.** A marked leukocytosis (WBC=158,000/μL) is evident.

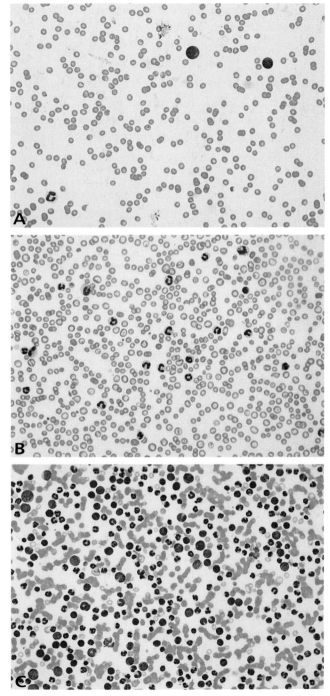

a mental image of the appearance of typical leukocytes of each cell line (neutrophil, eosinophil, lymphocyte, monocyte) (Figure 3-6).

- Evaluate the red cells for evidence of polychromasia, anisocytosis, hypochromasia, poikilocytosis, etc.
- Note any unusual findings (atypical cells, parasites).
▶ Oil immersion magnification.
- Examine erythrocytes and confirm observations made at low magnification (size, shape, color, abnormalities and any inclusions).
- Examine platelet morphology and distribution; estimate relative number.
- Examine leukocyte morphology (abnormalities and inclusions).
- Perform differential leukocyte count if not using automated equipment.
- If using automated equipment, estimate the differential count and compare to that reported by the instrument; this serves as an in-clinic quality control check!

# Quantitative Methods
## Packed Cell Volume (microhematocrit)

▶ Microhematocrits are accurate and repeatable. Instrumentation and supplies are inexpensive and suitable for all practices (Figure 3-7).

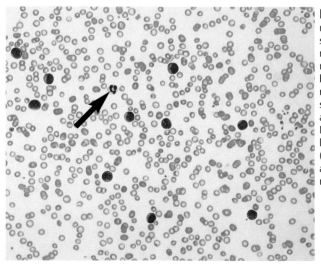

**Figure 3-6** Major abnormalities can be detected by scanning a smear. The majority of leukocytes in a normal canine or feline blood film should be segmented neutrophils. In this smear, most of the WBCs are large mononuclear cells. Note that these cells are larger than a neutrophil (arrow) and are most likely atypical lymphocytes or neoplastic cells.

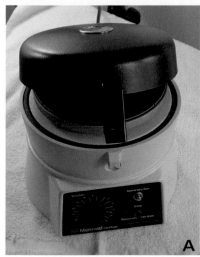

**Figure 3-7** Microhematocrit centrifuge and **(A)** card reader **(B)** to measure PCV. The microhematocrit centrifuge produces accurate measurements of circulating RBC mass and provides an opportunity to assess abnormalities in plasma color and to measure the total protein concentration by refractometry.

▶ High speed centrifugation is used to separate cells from plasma.

▶ The major source of error is trying to save time by not allowing the sample to spin the full amount of time. This produces an overestimate of the PCV because the plasma and cells are not fully separated.

▶ Hematocrits may also be computed and reported by in-clinic automated analyzers.

▶ The appearance of plasma in hematocrit tubes also can provide important information. Icterus, hemolysis, and lipemia may all be detected (Figure 3-8).

## Total Plasma Protein

▶ Total plasma protein can be measured easily by refractometry (Figure 3-9). For dogs and cats, the reference range is generally between 5.5 g/dl and 7.5 g/dl.

▶ Low total protein values reflect one of the following abnormalities
  – Protein losing nephropathy (characterized by proteinuria).
  – Protein losing enteropathy (usually associated with chronic weight loss and diarrhea).
  – Loss of lymph (check for pleural or peritoneal effusion).
  – Chronic or severe blood loss (check hematocrit!).
  – Lack of protein production by the liver.

▶ Elevated protein values reflect either hemoconcentration or increased globulin production.

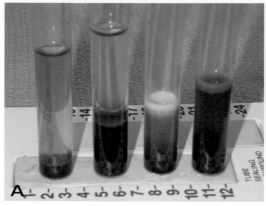
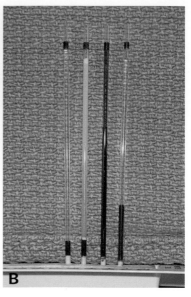

**Figure 3-8** Abnormal plasma colors in canine plasmas. In the large blood tubes **(A)**, from left to right, icterus, normal plasma, lipemia with hemolysis, and hemolysis are noted. Abnormal plasma colors in microhematocrit tubes **(B)** are more difficult to observe because of their small diameters. Icterus, lipemia, hemolysis, and normal plasma are displayed left to right. The first two samples are animals that were anemic. Note the markedly reduced PCV.

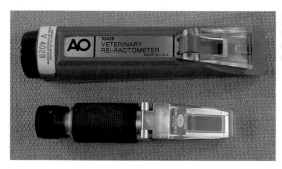

**Figure 3-9** Hand held refractometers can be easily used to determine total plasma protein as well as urine specific gravity.

- Hemoconcentration can cause elevations in red cell parameters, concentrated urine specific gravity, and elevations in serum electrolytes.
- Increased globulin production is most commonly associated with inflammation; an inflammatory leukogram is generally present.

▶ Evaluation of serum protein and serum albumin levels are useful in further clarifying the interpretation of plasma protein abnormalities.

## *Hemoglobin Concentration*

▶ Hand held hemoglobinometers provide a simple and rapid method to estimate hemoglobin concentration if automated equipment is not available.

▶ Some in-clinic chemistry analyzers measure hemoglobin in whole blood samples electrochemically.

## *Manual Cell Counts (Figure 3-10)*
▶ Microscopic counting of red and white cells is the oldest and most time-consuming method of determining blood cell counts.
▶ Microscope and special slide (hemocytometer) are required.
  – The hemocytometer is calibrated to hold a known volume of fluid between the cover slip and a grid etched on the slide
  – Can also used for counting cells in other body fluids and effusions.
▶ Dilution of blood
  – Different dilutions for red and white cell counts are necessary.
  – For white cell counts, erythrocytes are lysed.
  – The Unopette® System (Becton Dickinson, Franklin Lakes, NJ) provides a convenient and reproducible system of pre-measured diluents (Figure 3-11).
▶ Red cell count
  – Red cells can be counted using a hemocytometer, but the margin of error is high even among skilled medical technologists.
  – Red cell counts themselves offer little additional information over the hematocrit. They are needed to calculate of red cell indices, but manual counts are generally too variable to yield reliable information.
▶ Reticulocyte count
  – Performed by counting at least 1,000 erythrocytes on a smear made with supravital (new methylene blue) stained blood.
  – The absolute reticulocyte count is determined by multiplying the red cell count times the percent of reticulocytes.
▶ Differential white cell count
  – The stained smear should be examined with the oil immersion lens.
  – 100-200 white cells are characterized by type. The larger the number counted, the smaller the margin of error.
    • Avoid areas where cells are overlapping or distorted.
    • Use a consistent method to scan the slide to ensure random sampling and avoid counting the same area twice.
  – The percent of each cell type is multiplied by the total white cell count to determine the absolute number of each leukocyte/μl.
    • Absolute numbers (not %) should always be used in evaluating the hemogram.

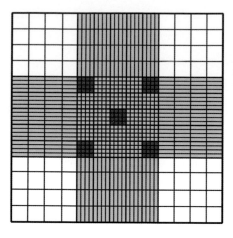

## Figure 3-10A

Hemocytometer grid lines. Erythrocyte and leukocyte count. Red = zones to be counted under high power for erythrocytes. White = zones to be counted under low power for leukocytes.

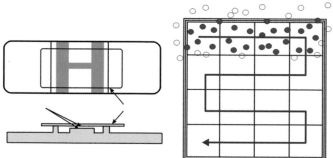

## Figure 3-10B

Left: The hemocytometer is designed to keep the coverglass 0.1 mm above the grid so that there is a known volume of fluid over each grid area. Right: The arrow indicates the direction in which the count should be made. Triple ruling: Cells touching top and left center lines are counted (shaded cells for the first row). Cells touching bottom and right center lines are not counted. Double ruling: Cells touching top and left outer lines are counted. Cells touching bottom and right inner lines are not counted.

*Reprinted with permission from Benjamin MM, outline of Veterinary Clinical Pathology, 3 ed., Ames, IA, the Iowa State University Press, 1978*

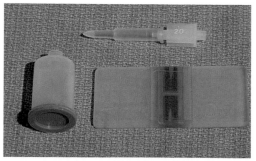

**Figure 3-11** Unopette® diluting pipette and reservoir for counting WBCs and platelets in a hemocytometer.

▶ Platelet count
- Can be performed using hemocytometer and ammonium oxalate diluent but it is difficult to achieve accuracy even among skilled medical technologists.
- Platelet count can be estimated from the blood smear.
  • 10-12 platelets per oil immersion field (100x nose piece objective) is an appropriate number in the dog and cat.
  • In the absence of obvious clumping, fewer than 10-12 platelets per 100x field suggests thrombocytopenia and indicates the need for a quantitative platelet count.

Advantages
▶ Manual counting is the least expensive in terms of equipment, supplies.
▶ Can be performed in mobile clinics.

Limitations
▶ Time consuming; most expensive in terms of professional staff time.
▶ Greatest variability/ unreliability in results.
- Inherent error is 20% or more, even among experienced technologists.
- Requires a high level of care and skill to produce accurate and precise results.

## Automated Cell Counters
▶ Several kinds and brands of electronic cell counters are now available for use in veterinary hospitals.
▶ All produce more accurate counts than manual methods and require less technician time.
- Compared to manual methods, a much larger number of cells are counted (several thousand) producing repeatable differentials and absolute counts.
▶ Some automated in-office equipment will produce partial or, more recently, complete differential counts.
- The most recently-introduced systems also produce accurate platelet and reticulocyte counts.
▶ In-office equipment offers the advantage of immediacy, producing results during the visit.
- It is therefore especially well suited to acute care and to pre-anesthetic and well-patient screening.

▶ Systems are of two types: semi-automated and fully automated.
  – Semi-automated equipment requires sample preparation (for example, dilution) by a technician; fully automated equipment performs all steps subsequent to obtaining the sample itself.
▶ All automated equipment must be properly maintained and periodically re-calibrated to produce accurate and consistent results.
  – Written standard operating procedures should be available and understood by all persons who will be operating the equipment.
  – The manufacturer's recommendations for instrument calibration, quality control, and maintenance should be followed closely. Establishing guidelines for in-clinic quality control is essential.
  – Instruments designed for analysis of human blood samples require modification and validation to produce accurate hemograms for other species.
▶ Each method has its strengths and limitations (see below); like all techniques in medicine, automated cell counting must be used intelligently.
  – The clinician should first rule out laboratory or collection artifact when the lab data are incongruent with the clinical assessment.

## Impedance (Figure 3-12)

▶ All impedance counters make use of Coulter principle.
▶ A dilute solution of cells in electrolyte solution is drawn through a small aperture between two electrodes.
▶ When a particle passes through the opening, it causes a change in electrical impedance and a measurable voltage pulse.
  – The magnitude of the voltage change is proportional to the size of the cell.
  – Voltage pulses are detected, analyzed and counted electronically.
▶ The red cell count actually includes both red and white cells, but because the proportion of white cells is usually small, the effect is insignificant unless the animal is simultaneously anemic and leukemic.
▶ Red cells are lysed in order to obtain a white cell count.
▶ Erythrocytes and platelets are differentiated on the basis of size (magnitude of the voltage change).

Advantages
▶ Faster and more effective use of staff time than manual methods.
▶ Newer models store calibration settings for different species.

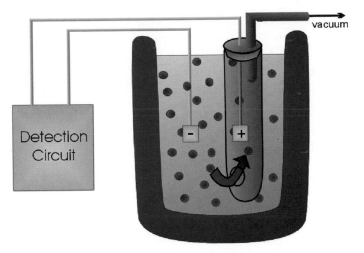

**Figure 3-12** Impedance counters rely on the Coulter principle. When a particle passes through a narrow orifice, it cause a change in the resistance. The magnitude of the change (corresponding to cell size) and the number (corresponding to the number of cells) are recorded by the detection circuit.

▶ Fully automated impedance counters are available for veterinary use that simultaneously perform RBC, WBC and platelet counts, determine mean corpuscular volume, and calculate hematocrit, MCHC and MCH.

▶ Some of the newer systems produce three-part differentials.

▶ Relatively inexpensive to operate and use.

Limitations

▶ Major limitation is the lack of any reticulocyte data.

▶ Major limitation is the inability to produce a complete differential count. Impedance counters group granulocytes into one catagory.

▶ Older models still require multiple step sample processing (dilution); red and white cells must be counted in separate steps.

▶ Relatively poor ability to differentiate among white cells and to differentiate white cells from nucleated RBCs.
  – WBC cell count must be corrected for nucleated RBCs.

▶ The overlap in size between feline platelets and erythrocytes leads to overestimates of the erythrocyte count and underestimates platelet numbers.

▶ Clumping of leukocytes leads to undercounting, and artifactual leukopenia.

▶ Only nuclear material is analyzed not cytoplasmic.

▶ Does not distinguish between bands and seperated neutrophils; consequntly a left shift cannot be determined from impedance data.

▶ Fibrin strands resulting from microclotting can plug the aperture and cause falsely decreased counts.

▶ Aggregates of platelets may be counted as white cells; this is especially problematic in cats.

▶ White cell counts are determined after lysing red cells; failure of RBCs to lyse completely produces falsely elevated white cell counts.
  – Erythrocytes with Heinz bodies don't lyse; hence, cats with large numbers of Heinz bodies may have falsely elevated WBC counts, hemoglobin measurement and the RBC indices (MCH, MCHC).
  – Polychromatic erythrocytes are more resistant to lysing and lead to falsely elevated WBC counts.

## Quantitative Buffy Coat (QBC) Analysis (Figure 3-13)

▶ Based on differential centrifugation
  – Under high speed centrifugation, blood separates into plasma, buffy coat and red cells.
  – The buffy coat itself is divided into layers based the relative density of the white cells and platelets; the platelets are the least dense and form a layer just beneath the plasma. Followed by monocytes and lymphocytes the granulocytes are the most dense of the white cells and come to rest immediately on top of the erythrocytes.

▶ Uses special acridine orange-coated tubes that include a cylindrical float with the same density as the buffy coat. When a tube is centrifuged, the float effectively reduces the diameter of the tube in the region of the buffy coat, causing it to spread along a greater length of the tube, enabling resolution of the various layers.

▶ The acridine orange stains nucleoproteins and other cellular components, which fluoresce when exposed to ultraviolet light.

▶ An automated reader (QBC® Vet Autoread, IDEXX Laboratories, Westbrook, Maine) scans the buffy coat layer and records the intensity of fluorescence produced by DNA and RNA/lipoproteins. Abrupt changes in slope are used to detect changes in cell type. The relative width of each band of fluorescence is used to calculate the population of cells.
  – The results and a graph of the pattern are printed out. The software is programmed to alert the operator of unexpected or uninterpretable results or patterns.

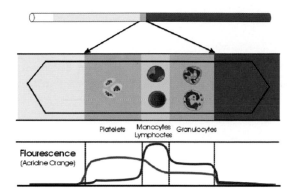

**Figure 3-13** The quantitative buffy coat (QBC) uses centrifugation to separate cells by density. A 'float' in the QBC tube reduces the volume of the lumen in the area of the buffy coat, causing the cells to be spread out over a greater distance. Cells types are differentiated by fluorescence in the presence of acridine orange.

Advantages
► The QBC is an efficient and economical way to screen blood samples.
► Instrument is simple to operate and relatively fast, producing results in about 7 minutes making it especially valuable for pre-anesthetic, acute care and in-office screening procedures.
► Hematocrit, hemoglobin, and white cell and platelet counts correlate well with reference methods.
► System flags abnormal or unexpected result.

Limitations
► The major limitation is the inability to produce a complete differential count. QBC cannot distinguish between lymphocytes and monocytes. Canine eosinophils inconsistently separated from lymphocytes and monocytes.
► Does not distinguish between bands and segmented neutrophils. The degree of left shift cannot be determined from the QBC data.
► Tends to underestimate frequency of leukopenia.
► Algorithms used to calculate RBC and WBC counts assume normal cell size and structure. They are thus invalidated by conditions such as microcytosis, hypochromasia, and cell immaturity. Assessment of a stained blood smear is essential to rule out conditions that could lead to inaccurate differential counts.

## Flow Cytometry (Figure 3-14)

- ▶ Laser flow cytometry is the newest and most accurate method of automated cell counting.
- ▶ Generally considered the gold standard in automated hematology
  - Used in most commercial laboratories, but until recently was cost-prohibitive for in-office use.
- ▶ A suspension of blood cells is broken into micro-droplets and passed through a laser beam.
- ▶ Cells absorb and scatter the laser light. Each cell type produces a characteristic "signature" depending on its size, nuclear configuration and cytoplasmic inclusions.
- ▶ The most sophisticated models generate a five-part differential, platelet count, reticulocyte count, and red cell indices.
- ▶ Fully automated models require no dilution or other sample preparation.
- ▶ Advanced units include particle standards in the diluent.

Advantages

- ▶ Because laser flow cytometry systems evaluate multiple parameters (nuclear and cytoplasmic material) of each cell or platelet, they produce more accurate and reliable counts than other methods.
- ▶ Clumped cells or platelets can be detected and ignored.
- ▶ Large platelets (frequently encountered in cats) can be distinguished from erythrocytes due to difference in light scattering caused by the platelet granules.
- ▶ Flow cytometers are able to rapidly count and categorize large numbers (>2,000) of erythrocytes which are needed to produce accurate and repeatable reticulocyte counts.

Limitations

- ▶ In some systems, light scattering from aggregates of granular platelets produces a pattern that can be miscounted as leukocytes (pseudoleukocytosis).
- ▶ Although recent breakthroughs in technology have reduced the cost so that these units are economically justified in most hospitals, they may not be economical in small practices or those that make minimal use of hematology.
- ▶ Examination of the blood film is still needed to detect abnormalities such as the presence of left shift, toxicity, reactive lymphocytes, blast cells, mast cells, microfilaria and red cell parasites.

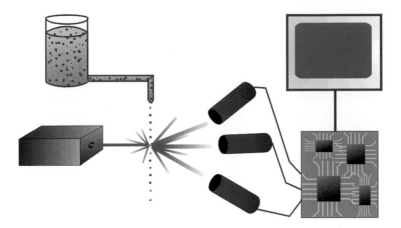

**Figure 3-14** Laser flow cytometry detects and counts individual cells in micro-droplets as they pass through a laser beam. Each cell type scatters the laser in a characteristic 'signature' based on its size, nucleus and cytoplasmic contents.

## *Commercial Laboratory*

▶ Many commercial laboratories offer hematology services at reasonable prices to veterinarians.

▶ Leading laboratories have state of the art equipment because they are able to amortize the cost over a very large number of samples.

▶ Counts are performed on automated equipment supplemented by microscopic examination by trained personnel.

Advantages

▶ Well-run laboratories have quality control programs to ensure accuracy.

▶ Films are evaluated by personnel who evaluate hundreds of smears daily. They are thus more likely to notice and diagnose rare and unusual abnormalities.

▶ Identification of bizarre or neoplastic cells is a job for an expert; unusual or highly abnormal samples should be sent to a laboratory with a board-certified veterinary clinical pathologist.

▶ Red cell parasites and inclusions can also be difficult to differentiate and should be sent for expert confirmation.

▶ Commercial laboratories can provide additional commentary on unusual findings and consultation with veterinary clinical pathologists.

Limitations

    ▶ The main drawback to the use of external laboratories is time; results are not usually available for several hours or until the next day.

       – Can be an issue for time-sensitive cases or pre-anesthetic screening.

       – Fresh blood smears shuld be prepared in-clinic and sent with EDTA samples is hematology is performed at reference laboratories.

       – Check with your reference laboratory and confirm that blood smears are at least scanned by trained professionals.

▶ Hematology is species specific. Some laboratories that do primarily human clinical pathology will accept veterinary samples, but this can lead to erroneous results.

       – Automated hematology equipment must be re-calibrated for each species or it will produce inaccurate results.

       – Likewise, persons evaluating blood smears must be familiar with species differences or they may mis-classify white blood cell types and may misinterpret normal variation as a disease condition.

       – Large laboratories have many technologists. Each technologist evaluates blood films somewhat differently. The veterinarian cannot assume that all slides are evaluated in the same way.

       – Always use a veterinary reference laboratory or one that is familiar with evaluating veterinary samples and has veterinary pathologists on staff.

# 4

# Erythrocytes

# OVERVIEW
## Production

Red blood cells (RBC) are produced in the bone marrow.

Numbers of circulating RBCs are affected by changes in plasma volume, rate of RBC destruction or loss, splenic contraction, erythropoietin (EPO) secretion, and the rate of bone marrow production.

A normal PCV is maintained by an endocrine loop that involves generation and release of erythropoietin (EPO) from the kidney in response to renal hypoxia.

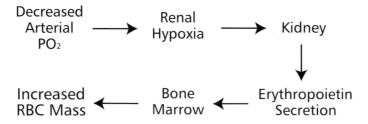

Erythropoietin stimulates platelet production as well as red cell production. However, erythropoietin **does not** stimulate white blood cell (WBC) production.

Erythropoiesis and RBC numbers are also affected by hormones from the adrenal cortex, thyroid, ovary, testis, and anterior pituitary.

## Destruction

Red cells have a finite circulating lifespan. In dogs, the average normal red cell circulates approximately 100 days. In cats, 85-90 days.

Since in health circulating red cell numbers remain fairly constant, approximately 1% of the circulating red cells of the dog are replaced daily (slightly higher percentage in the cat). The new cells are young and morphologically distinct (large, polychromatophilic – see morphology section).

Effete red cells are phagocytized and metabolized by the macrophages of spleen, bone marrow, and liver. Iron is preserved for reutilization.

## Function

The primary function of the red cell is to carry oxygen to tissue cells and to carry carbon dioxide away.

To facilitate this exchange, red cells consist essentially of gas-carrying soluble protein (hemoglobin) surrounded by a protective cell membrane.

The fluidity of normal red cells allow them to traverse tortuous capillary beds leading to close approximation of red cells with tissue cells. This in turn makes gaseous exchange efficient.

## Physiology

Red cell physiology is geared to facilitate function and protect red cell integrity.

The primary red cell metabolic pathway is anaerobic glycolysis. The glycolytic pathway allows the cell to produce energy to maintain membrane stability with minimal utilization of oxygen.

The red cell also has metabolic pathways (hexose monophosphate shunt and methemoglobin reductase) which protect hemoglobin from oxidation. Oxidation of hemoglobin leads to methemoglobinemia and/or Heinz body formation.

Cat hemoglobin is more susceptible to oxidation than dog hemoglobin because it contains a high percentage of sulfur-containing amino acids which are easily oxidized. Therefore, Heinz body formation and Heinz body hemolytic anemia occurs more readily in cats than dogs.

# MORPHOLOGY
## Normal Morphology: Dog

Shape: biconcave disc with prominent central pallor (Figure 4-1)

Size: 6.0-7.0 $\mu$

Rouleaux formation (stacking): moderate (Figure 4-2)

Polychromatophils (bluish-red immature erythrocytes): comprise approximately 1% of total red cell population (Figures 4-3 and 4-4)

Polychromatophils correspond to reticulocytes in new methylene blue stained preparations (Figure 4-5)

Howell-Jolly bodies are deeply staining nuclear remnants found in red cells. These inclusions are rare in normal dogs (Figure 4-6).

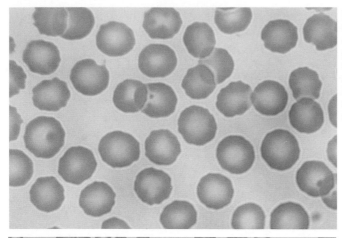

**Figure 4-1**
Canine blood, normal erythrocyte morphology. Canine RBCs are all about the same size, shape, and color, and have a prominent area of central pallor (100x).

**Figure 4-2**
Canine blood, rouleaux formation. RBCs are arranged in overlapping chains (60x).

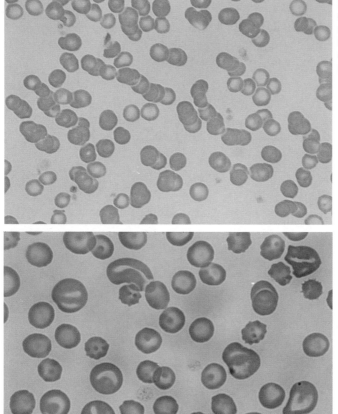

**Figure 4-3**
Canine blood. Regenerative anemia. Immature RBCs are visible as larger erythrocytes that have blue-grey cytoplasm. These cells are termed macrocytic polychromatophilic erythrocytes (100x).

## Figure 4-4
Canine blood. Iron deficiency anemia. Hypochromia and poikilocytosis are evident. Hypochromic RBCs have a large area of central pallor due to reduced hemoglobin content. The polychromatophilic RBC (arrow) in this field has a vacuolated or moth-eaten cytoplasm. Compare these cells with those in Figure 4-3 (100x).

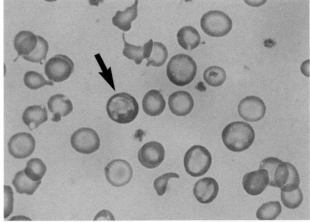

## Figure 4-5
Canine blood. New methylene blue stain. Reticulocytes are visible as pale yellow cells with basophilic precipitates of RNA (100x).

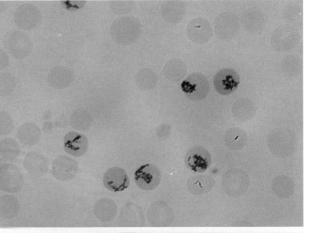

## Figure 4-6
Canine blood, Howell Jolly body. Small basophilic round inclusion in the RBC cytoplasm (arrow) is a remnant of a nucleus (100x).

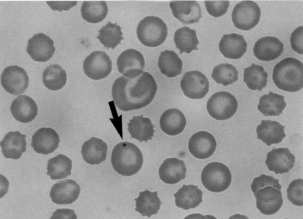

# Normal Morphology: Cat

Shape: biconcave disc with minimal central pallor (Figure 4-7)

Size: 5.5-6.0 $\mu$

Rouleaux formation: marked

Polychromatophils: comprise 1.5-2.0% of total red cell population (Figure 4-8)

Howell-Jolly bodies: occasional; more common than in dogs.

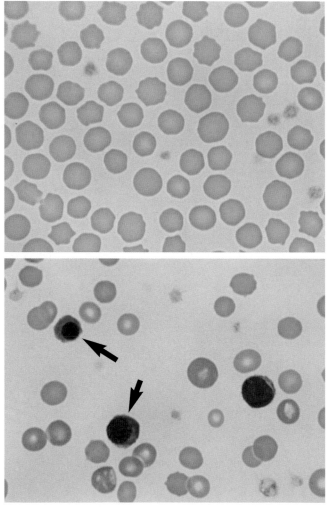

**Figure 4-7**
Feline blood.
Normal erythrocyte morphology. Feline RBCs are smaller than dog erythrocytes, exhibit a slight amount of crenation, and have a minimal area of central pallor (100x).

**Figure 4-8**
Feline blood.
Regenerative anemia. Immature RBCs are visible as larger erythrocytes that have blue-grey cytoplasm. These cells are termed macrocytic polychromatophilic erythrocytes. Two NRBCs (arrows) are noted and are smaller than a lymphocyte (100x).

# Morphology in Disease

Anisocytosis – variation in red cell size (Figure 4-9).

- ► Macrocytes – large red cells
- ► Microcytes – small red cells

Polychromasia – increased numbers of polychromatophils on the blood film.

Hypochromasia – decreased hemoglobin concentration. Hypochromic red cells have enlarged areas of central pallor (Figure 4-10).

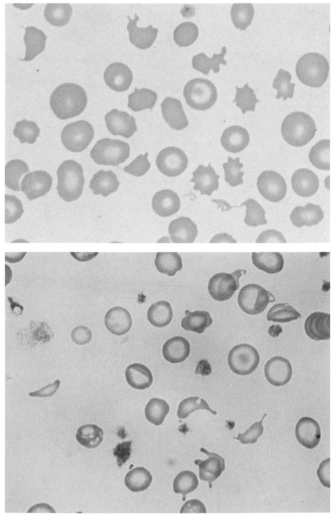

**Figure 4-9**
Canine blood. Marked anisocytosis and poikilocytosis are present due to macrocytic cells, spherocytes, schistocytes, acanthocytes and microcytes (100x). See subsequent figures for indentification of specific poikilocytes.

**Figure 4-10**
Canine blood. Numerous poikilocytes, marked hypochromia, and microcytosis are evident. Platelets are numerous and enlarged. These changes are usually associated with iron deficiency secondary to chronic hemorrhage (100x).

Poikilocytosis–the presence of abnormally shaped red cells.

▶ Acanthocytes – red cells with 2-10 blunt elongate finger-like surface projections (Figure 4-11).

▶ Spherocytes – small round red cells that stain intensely and lack central pallor (Figure 4-12).

▶ Elliptocytes – oval erythrocytes.

▶ Dacryocytes – tear-drop shaped erythrocytes.

▶ Stomatocytes – cup-shaped erythrocytes (Figure 4-12).

▶ Heinz bodies – precipitates of oxidized hemoglobin. Often recognized as nose-like projections from the red cell surface (Figures 4-13 and 4-14).

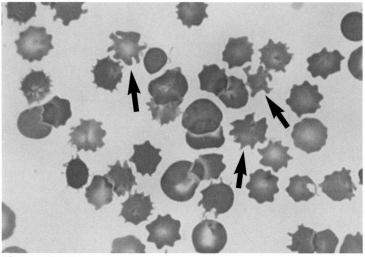

**Figure 4-11**
Canine blood. The poikilocytes in this blood smear have irregular membrane projections that have rounded tips. These cells are called acanthocytes (arrows) and represent an in vivo alteration rather than an artifact. Acanthocytes are frequently associated with hemangiosarcoma in the liver. A few spherocytes are also noted. (100x).

▶ Eccentrocytes – red cells with hemoglobin concentrated at one pole with an unstained area at the other pole (Figures 4-15 and 4-16).

▶ Schistocytes – irregularly shaped, often roughly triangular, red cell fragments (Figure 4-17).

▶ Burr cells – elongated red cells with ruffled margins (also termed echino elliptocytes).

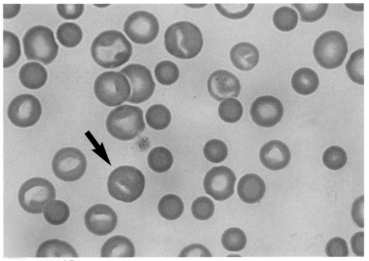

## Figure 4-12

Canine blood. Regenerative anemia with spherocytes. Anisocytosis is due to macrocytic cells and spherocytes, which are smaller than normal and lack central pallor. Spherocytes are associated with hemolytic anemias due to immune disease or fragmentation. The polychromatophilic RBC with a rod-shaped area of central pallor (arrow) is a stomatocyte (100x).

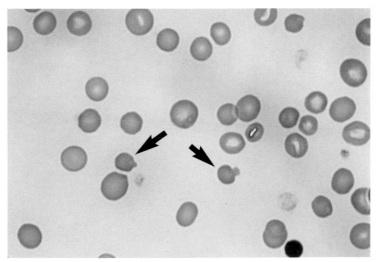

## Figure 4-13

Feline blood. Heinz body hemolytic anemia. Morphologic evidence of regenerative anemia is present as anisocytosis and polychromasia. Smaller RBCs (arrows) have singular rounded membrane projections that are Heinz bodies. These inclusions are caused by oxidative injury due to drugs, toxic plants, certain chemicals, and metabolic diseases. Heinz bodies can be seen in cats that are clinically normal and not anemic (100x).

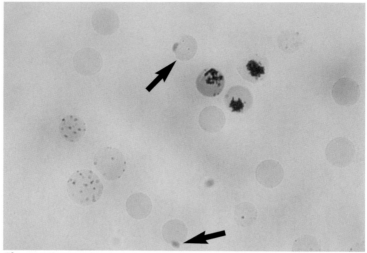

**Figure 4-14**
Feline blood. New methylene blue stain. Heinz bodies are noted on the edge of RBCs as turquoise inclusions (arrows). Aggregate and punctate reticulocytes can also be seen. Aggregate reticulocytes have definite clumps of RNA precipitate in the RBC cytoplasm. Punctate reticulocytes left of center have numerous small individual granules of RNA precipitate. When counting reticulocytes for the absolute reticulocyte count, only aggregate reticulocytes are enumerated to assess the regenerative response (100x).

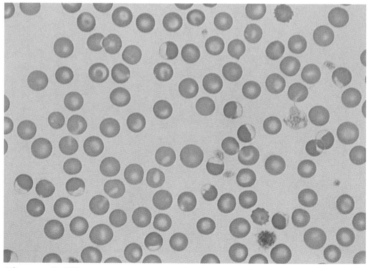

**Figure 4-15**
Canine blood. Hemolytic disease. RBC with eccentric hemoglobin staining can be seen (eccentrocytes). Very little evidence of anisocytosis or polychromasia can be seen (60x).

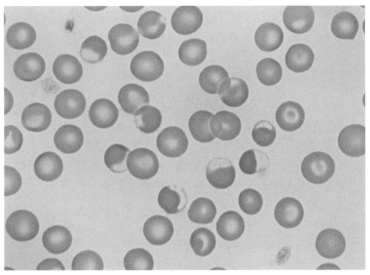

## Figure 4-16
Canine blood. Hemolytic disease. Numerous eccentrocytes or "blister cells" are seen. These cells have an eccentric displacement of hemoglobin because opposing sides of the RBC membrane have fused due to oxidative injury. Causes of this change are identical to those that produce Heinz bodies (100x).

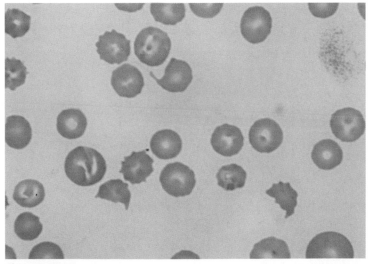

## Figure 4-17
Canine blood. Schistocytes. Fragmentation of RBCs results in the formation of schistocytes. These cells are formed when RBCs are sheared by convoluted vascular channels, intravascular fibrin deposition, or excessive turbulence. The RBCs have sharp cuts in the cell margin that produce membrane tags and cells that have a helmet shape (100x).

# Artifacts

Crenation: the presence of red cells covered by short spiky surface projections (Figure 4-18).

▶ Crenation is the most common artifactual change seen in blood films.

▶ Crenation can be confused with acanthocytic change.

▶ Crenation is more prominent in films made from EDTA blood.

▶ Crenation is differentiated from true poikilocytosis in that crenation affects all the red cells in a given area of the film whereas true poikilocytosis affects only scattered red cells on the blood film.

Refractory "bubbles" on the surface of red cells (Figure 4-19).

▶ Refractory areas on the red cell surface are most commonly seen when blood films are stained while still wet.

▶ These "bubbles" probably represent gas being trapped in the specimen as it escapes from the red cells.

Stain precipitate

▶ Aggregates of stain precipitate are commonly observed on Romanowsky (Wright's, Diff Quik) stained slides.

▶ Stain precipitate along the margins of red cells must be differentiated from Hemobartonella organisms (Figures 4-20 and 4-21).

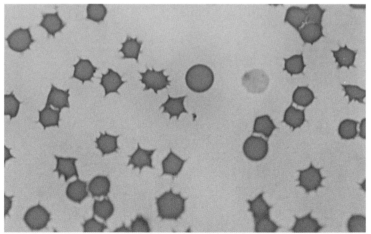

**Figure 4-18**
Short regular membrane projections with sharp points represent an artifact in RBC morphology called crenation. This change can occur due to a delay between collection of blood and smear preparation, or due to a drying artifact (100x).

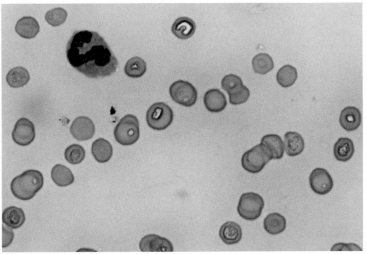

**Figure 4 19**
Feline blood. Refractile artifact. Air bubbles trapped in the area of central pallor produces a refractile rounded structure that may be confused with an RBC inclusion. These structures "jewel" as the fine focus is moved and can be seen in a plane of focus that is beyond the RBC membrane (100x).

▶ Stain precipitate must also be differentiated from basophilic stippling (Figure 4-22).

Over-staining of red cells
  ▶ Slides which have been exposed to formalin fumes will have an overall greenish discoloration when stained.  It will be difficult to recognize polychromasia in such preparation.
  ▶ Slides which are exposed too long to the basophilic (blue) component of Romanowsky stains will also be over-stained, making evaluation of polychromasia difficult to impossible.

Scratching the preparation
  ▶ Wiping or blotting the surface of a blood film with a tissue or lens paper to dry it or remove oil will leave scratches. This should be avoided.
  ▶ Scratches are seen microscopically as linear disruptions of cells, particularly red cells.
  ▶ Cells broken in this manner may be mistaken for schistocytes.

Pseudothrombocytopenia
  ▶ Clumping of platelets can falsely decrease the platelet counts especially in cats (Figure 4-23).

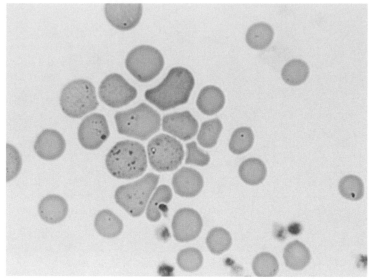

**Figure 4-20**
Canine blood. Granular artifact. Stain precipitate can sometimes adhere to RBCs and produce the appearance of a parasite or inclusion. These granules vary in size and do not resemble any of the usual canine RBC parasites. If the focus were adjusted, this material would appear to "jewel" or be refractile (100x).

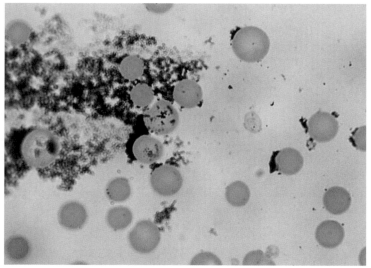

**Figure 4-21**
Feline blood. Precipitated stain. Basophilic granular material that obscures the RBCs is stain precipitate. This material is sometimes mistaken for bacteria or RBC parasites (100x).

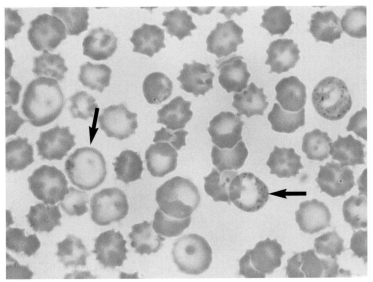

## Figure 4-22

Canine blood. Basophilic stippling. Several of the RBCs have small fine basophilic granules in the cytoplasm (arrows). Basophilic stippling can be seen in dogs and cats with severe regenerative anemias or in dogs with lead poisoning. In the latter disease, stippling is associated with an inappropriate release of NRBCs (100x).

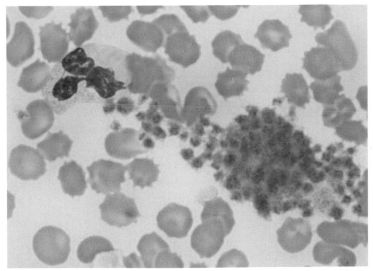

## Figure 4-23

Canine blood, platelet clump. Platelet clumping is usually a collection artifact that can produce a false decrease in platelet count. This is especially a problem in cats. Blood smears should be examined for aggregates of platelets when the electronic platelet count is low (100x).

# QUANTITY
## Anemia

Decreased red cell mass is anemia.

Anemias are classified as regenerative or nonregenerative based on bone marrow responsiveness.

### Regenerative Anemia

Regenerative anemias are anemias where marrow red cell production is increased to the point that red cell mass will eventually be returned to normal.

▶ Increased polychromatophils (young red cells – see morphology) in the peripheral circulation is the reflection of increased production on routinely stained blood films.

▶ The first step in differentiating regenerative from nonregenerative anemia is evaluation of the blood film.

Whenever increased polychromasia is seen on routine blood films, reticulocyte counts are warranted.

Reticulocyte counts of greater than 80,000/$\mu$l indicate regeneration.

Regenerative anemias are either the result of blood loss or hemolysis.

### Regenerative Anemia: Blood Loss / Hemorrhage

History, clinical signs, and physical examination often point to the source of blood loss.

In general, blood loss anemias are less responsive than hemolytic anemia. The main reason is that when blood loss occurs, iron is lost from the body and iron is needed for hemoglobin synthesis.

If blood loss is severe or chronic, iron depletion and/or iron deficiency can occur, resulting in a nonregenerative anemia.

The nonregenerative anemia of iron deficiency is often microcytic (small red cell size) and hypochromic (reduced hemoglobin). A description and illustration of iron deficiency anemia is found on page 59.

Since loss of blood involves loss of plasma protein as well as loss of cells, blood loss anemias may also have reduced plasma protein, serum protein, albumin, and globulin levels.

As a general guideline, absolute reticulocyte counts between 80,000/$\mu$l and 200,000/$\mu$l can indicate either blood loss or hemolysis.

▶ As reticulocyte counts elevate above 200,000/$\mu$l, hemolysis should be suspected.

## Regenerative Anemias: Hemolytic Disease

Hemolytic anemia occurs when the circulating red cell lifespan is reduced due to increased rates of RBC distruction.

▶ Hemolysis is the result either of a defect in the red cells (inherent or acquired) or a defect in the microvasculature through which the red cells circulate.

Hemolysis can occur intravascularly (while the red cells are circulating) or extravascularly.

▶ Extravascular hemolysis involves the destruction and removal of damaged red cells by the macrophages of the spleen and liver.

▶ Many hemolytic anemias have elements of both intravascular and extravascular lysis.

Hemoglobinemia and/or hemoglobinuria are seen only in severe cases of intravascular hemolysis

Icterus can be seen in either intravascular or extravascular hemolytic anemia.

Because hemolytic anemias are associated with red cell defects, red cell morphologic alterations often are associated with specific causes of hemolytic anemia. The common hemolytic anemias of the dog and cat are listed, described, and illustrated below.

### Hemolytic Disease: Immune-Mediated Hemolytic Anemia (IMHA)

▶ Occurs in both dogs and cats

▶ Pathogenesis:
  – Red cells become coated with antibodies as they circulate (Figure 4-24)
  – Antibody-coated red cells either lyse intravascularly (due to complement fixation) or are removed by macrophages in the liver and spleen.

▶ Antibodies may be directed against the red cells themselves (autoimmune hemolytic anemia) or against foreign antigens.

▶ Among the conditions which can cause immune-mediated hemolytic disease are:
  – Heartworm disease
  – Lymphoma
  – Lupus erythematosus
  – Drug-induced immune mediated hemolysis

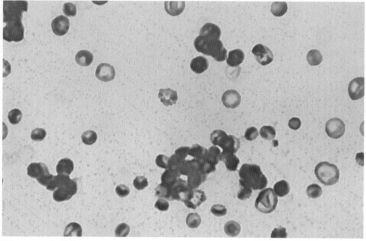

**Figure 4-24**
Canine blood. RBC agglutination. Branching chains of RBCs form clusters in three areas of the field. Agglutination of RBCs occurs when antibodies cause bridging between adjacent cells (100x).

▶ The morphologic hallmark of immune-mediated hemolytic anemia is the presence of significant numbers of spherocytes (Figures 4-25 and 4-26).

▶ Spherocytes are red cells with the following characteristics (Figure 4-26):
  – Small
  – Round
  – Stain intensely
  – Lack central pallor

▶ Ghost cells may also be present (Figures 4-25 and 4-27)

▶ Whenever blood film morphology suggests immune hemolysis (regenerative anemia with spherocytes), a Coomb's test (direct antiglobulin test) can be run for confirmation.

▶ The Coomb's test must be run with species specific Coomb's reagent or false positives can occur.

▶ False negative Coomb's tests are also common; these can be reduced in number by requesting that the laboratory run the test with serial dilutions of Coomb's reagent.

▶ The positive endpoint of the Coomb's test is agglutination.
  – Autoagglutination is seen in some cases of immune-mediated hemolysis (Figure 4-24).
  – If autoagglutination is present, the diagnosis of immune hemolysis is confirmed without running the Coomb's test.

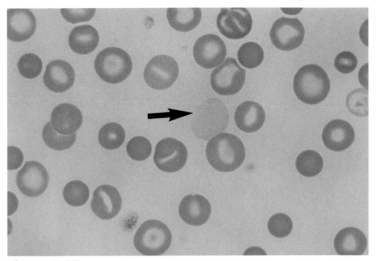

**Figure 4-25**

Canine blood. Spherocytosis. The smaller RBCs that lack central pallor are spherocytes. These cells are frequent in dogs with immune-mediated hemolytic disease. They can also occur in fragmentation hemolysis. A ghost RBC (arrow) is noted in the center of the field and suggests some degree of intravascular lysis (100x).

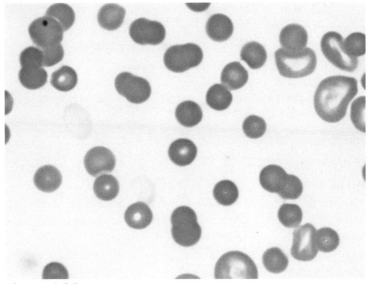

**Figure 4-26**

Spherocytosis. If this were a feline blood smear, the RBC morphology would indicate regenerative anemia. The small RBC without central pallor would represent normal feline erythrocytes. However, this is canine blood and the small RBCs without central pallor are spherocytes. This dog has a marked spherocytosis due to immune-mediated hemolytic disease (100x).

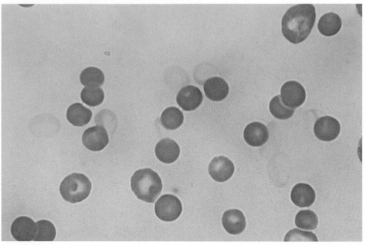

**Figure 4-27**
Canine blood, RBC ghosts. Several RBCs are noted that have almost no hemoglobin within their cytoplasm. Ghost RBCs usually indicate intravascular lysis of RBC which can occur with immune-mediated disease, Heinz body hemolysis, or with fragmentation injury (100x).

► Autoagglutination on blood films is seen as three-dimensional clumping of erythrocytes. This may be confused with rouleaux formation.

► Autoagglutination can be distinguished from rouleaux by preparing and examining a saline-diluted wet preparation.
  - Place 1 drop of EDTA-blood on a slide.
  - Add 2 drops of isotonic saline.
  - Coverslip and examine. If clumping is present, autoagglutination is confirmed.

## Hemolytic Disease: Heinz Body Anemia

► Occurs in dogs and cats

► Pathogenesis:
  - Circulating oxidants act on red cell hemoglobin at two primary sites: the sulfhydryl containing amino acids in globin, and the iron moiety.
  - Oxidation of globin leads to precipitation and the formation of Heinz bodies.
  - Oxidation of iron leads to methemoglobinemia.
  - Methemoglobinemia and Heinz bodies may occur in the same patient but one form is generally predominant.
  - Heinz body formation is most prevalent and easiest to recognize.

▶ Most cases of Heinz body hemolytic anemia are the result of ingestion of oxidizing substances such as onions or the action of oxidizing drugs such as acetaminophen (Figure 4-28).

▶ Heinz bodies are precipitates of oxidized hemoglobin.
  – They often become fixed to the red cell membrane and are recognized as nose-like projections on the red cell surface.
  – Cells from which Heinz bodies have been removed (torn away) may also be observed; these are known as bite cells.

▶ Eccentrocytes are also commonly observed in Heinz body hemolytic anemia.
  – Eccentrocytes are red cells which lack central pallor.
  – All of the hemoglobin is concentrated at one pole of the cell.
  – At the other pole is a small area of unstained cytoplasm bound by a distinct cell membrane.

▶ Eccentrocytes form when oxidation of the red cell membrane occurs. This leads to fusion of opposing sites on the red cell membrane which pushes the hemoglobin peripherally.

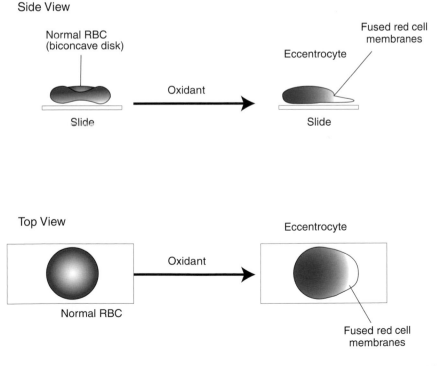

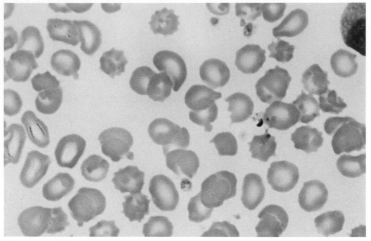

**Figure 4-28**
Canine blood. Heinz bodies. Round membrane projections on most of the RBCs are Heinz bodies. This dog ate onions, which can cause oxidative injury and Heinz body formation (100x).

► In routine blood films, Heinz bodies have the same staining characteristics as hemoglobin.

► In new methylene blue stained films, Heinz bodies are turquoise (Figure 4-29).

► Cat hemoglobin is more susceptible to oxidant damage than dog hemoglobin.

 – Cats are therefore more susceptible to Heinz body hemolysis.

 – Furthermore, Heinz bodies can be seen in large numbers in the absence of hemolytic anemia in certain metabolic conditions in cats (eg, diabetes mellitus, liver disease, hyperthyroidism, etc.).

► The diagnosis of Heinz body hemolytic anemia in cats requires the demonstration of large numbers of Heinz bodies **and** the presence of a significant regenerative anemia.

► In dogs, if Heinz bodies are present, Heinz body hemolytic disease is confirmed.

## Hemolytic Disease: Feline Haemobartonellosis

► Caused by *Haemobartonella felis*

► *H. felis* organisms are recognized on the red cell surface as either chains of small (1 $\mu$) basophilic rods or ring forms (Figure 4-30 and 4-31).

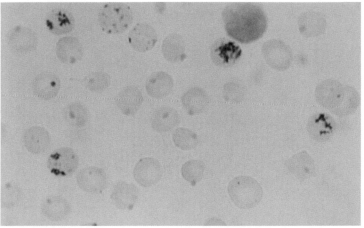

**Figure 4-29**
Canine blood. New methylene blue stain. Heinz bodies are noted as turquoise inclusions on the edge of the RBC membranes. Reticulocytes are also present (100x).

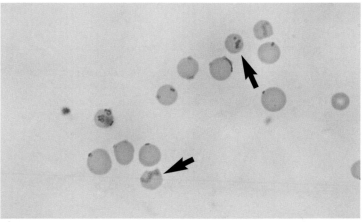

**Figure 4-30**
Feline blood. *Haemobartonella felis*. Blood smear from an anemic cat reveals the rod and coccoid forms of *Haemobartonella felis*. Ring forms (arrows) can be seen on the RBC surface in small groups (100x).

▶ Organisms must be differentiated from stain precipitate (Figure 4-20) and *Cytauxzoon felis* (Figure 4-32).

▶ Feline haemobartonellosis can occur as a primary disease or secondary to other immunosuppressive disorders such as FeLV infection, FIV infection, or FIP infection.

▶ Primary haemobartonellosis presents as a typical regenerative hemolytic anemia. Organisms appear intermittently in large numbers on peripheral erythrocytes.

▶ Secondary haemobartonellosis often presents as a severe nonregenerative anemia.

▶ Both primary and secondary haemobartonellosis may have an immune-mediated component and be Coomb's positive.

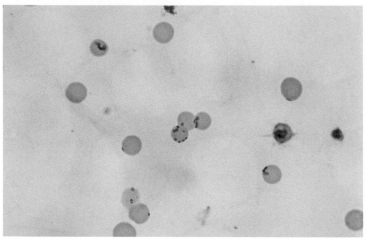

**Figure 4-31**
Feline blood. *Haemobartonella felis.* RBC density on the smear is reduced due to severe anemia. In this area of the smear, Haemobartonella organisms can be seen as basophilic rings on the RBC surface. These parasites produce hemolytic anemia by causing RBCs to be phagocytozed by macrophages (100x).

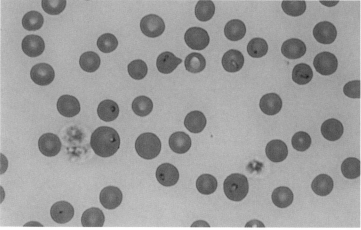

**Figure 4-32**
Feline blood. *Cytauxzoon felis.* This is an intracellular protozoan parasite of wild and domestic cats. In domestic cats, the parasite causes a nonregenerative anemia with round, oval, or safety pin shaped basophilic parasites in RBCs. (100x).

## Hemolytic Disease: Canine Haemobartonellosis

Less common than in cats

Caused by *Haemobartonella canis*

*H. canis* organisms form multiple chains on the red cell surface. Individual organisms are larger and easier to see than *H. felis* (Figure 4-33).

Canine haemobartonellosis generally presents as a true regenerative hemolytic anemia. However, it usually occurs secondarily to splenectomy or immunosuppressive events such as chemotherapy.

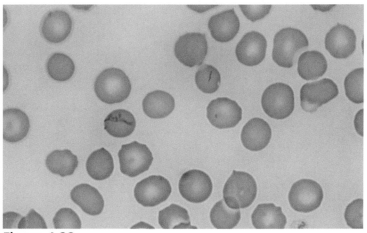

**Figure 4-33**
Canine blood. *Haemobartonella canis*. Long chains of small basophilic coccoid organisms are noted on the surface of two RBCs. In one cell, a double chain, or "bow string" form, is present. These organisms cause mild hemolytic anemia in dogs following splenectomy, or in association with immunosupression (100x).

## Hemolytic Disease: Canine Babesiosis

▶ Tick-borne protozoal disease of dogs.

▶ The causative agent is *Babesia canis* (Figure 4-34) or *Babesia gibsoni* (Figure 4-35).

▶ Babesiosis is a true intravascular hemolytic anemia, often characterized by hemoglobinemia and hemoglobinuria.

▶ Babesiosis may also have an immune-mediated component and be Coomb's positive.

▶ Babesia are recognized on peripheral blood films as intra-erythrocytic teardrop shaped organisms measuring approximately 1.5 (*B. gibsoni*) to 3 μ (*B. canis*) in length. Up to four organisms may be seen in a parasitized cell.

► As with haemobartonella organisms, prevalence of Babesia organisms in the blood film is cyclic.

## Hemolytic Disease: Pyruvate Kinase Deficiency (PK)

► Pyruvate kinase is an enzyme in the glycolytic pathway essential to the production of energy (ATP).

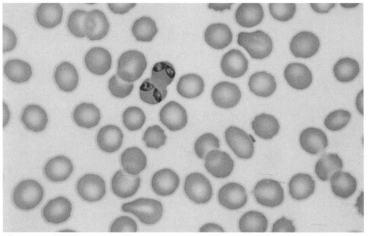

**Figure 4-34**
Canine blood. *Babesia canis*. Pairs of pyriform intracellular protozoal organisms are consistent with *Babesia canis* organisms. This parasite causes hemolysis by intravascular and extravascular RBC destruction (100x).

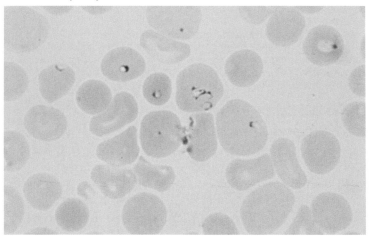

**Figure 4-35**
Canine blood. *Babesia gibsoni*. Round, oval, or elongate protozoal organisms that vary in size are present in several RBCs. An eccentric nuclear structure is visible in some organisms. This parasite was endemic in parts of Asia and is now present in North America (120x).

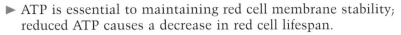

▶ ATP is essential to maintaining red cell membrane stability; reduced ATP causes a decrease in red cell lifespan.

▶ PK deficiency is a heritable hemolytic condition described in Beagles and Basenjis. It is present from the time of birth and usually recognized clinically by 3 years of age.

▶ In its early phases, pyruvate kinase deficiency induced hemolysis may present as compensated hemolysis. The blood film shows marked regeneration but the patient may not be anemic.

▶ Anemia develops as the patient ages. In late phases of the disease, the bone marrow apparently becomes exhausted and may become scarred (myelofibrosis). At this point, the anemia is non-regenerative and terminal. There is no treatment for this condition.

▶ PK deficiency hemolysis has been described as nonspherocytic hemolysis (Figure 4-36).
  – In some cases, spheroechinocytes can be found scattered on blood films of affected animals, but this is not a constant finding.
  – Spheroechinocytes are smaller than normal, lack central pallor, and are covered by short sharp spiky surface projections.

▶ Diagnosis can be confirmed by measuring red cell PK levels.

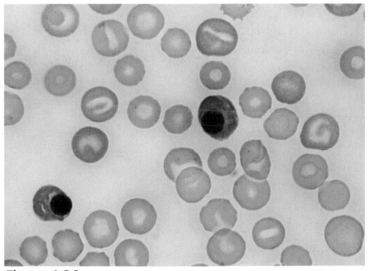

**Figure 4-36**
Canine blood. PK deficiency. Pyruvate kinase deficiency causes a chronic hemolytic anemia. RBC lifespan is decreased due to a metabolic defect in RBC metabolism. An intense regenerative response is present characterized by marked polychromasia, anisocytosis, macrocytosis, and NRBCs (100x).

### Hemolytic Disease: Phosphofructokinase (PFK) Deficiency

▶ PFK is also a glycolytic enzyme essential to ATP production.

▶ Reduced ATP in RBC's leads to shortened red cell lifespan (hemolysis).

▶ PFK deficiency is a rare heritable hemolytic condition described only in Springer Spaniels.

▶ There is no distinctive morphologic footprint for PFK deficiency.

▶ Diagnosis is confirmed through analysis of red cell enzyme levels.

### Hemolytic Disease: Mechanical Hemolysis

▶ There are two distinct mechanisms for mechanical hemolysis:

- Normal red cells are forced to traverse abnormally tortuous capillary beds. This leads to intravascular shearing of red cells and shortened red cell lifespan. This is termed microangiopathic hemolysis. Common causes include:
  - Glomerulonephritis
  - DIC
  - Hemangiosarcoma
- Normal red cells are exposed to turbulent blood flow in large vessels. Examples include:
  - Heartworm disease
  - Traumatic disruption of red cells in heart disease

▶ The morphologic footprint of mechanical hemolysis is the schistocyte. Schistocytes are small irregularly shaped red cell fragments.

## Non-regenerative Anemia

Non-regenerative anemias are the result of either ineffective erythropoiesis (maturation defect anemias) or reduced production of red cells (hypoproliferative anemias).

Maturation defect anemias can generally be suspected from changes in the peripheral blood.

With a few notable exceptions, hypoproliferative anemias require bone marrow examination for diagnosis.

## Maturation Defect Anemias

These anemias have non-regenerative peripheral blood patterns (absence of increased polychromasia/reticulocytosis) but erythroid hyperplasia in the bone marrow.

Red cell production is therefore ineffective in that the increased red cell production in the marrow is not reflected in the peripheral blood.

Maturation defect anemias are classified as either nuclear maturation defect anemias or cytoplasmic maturation defect anemias.

### Maturation Defect Anemias: Nuclear Defect (megaloblastic anemias)

▶ The principal problem in these anemias is an acquired bone marrow defect in which precursor nuclei of all cell lines fail to mature and divide normally while cytoplasmic maturation proceeds unimpaired (Figures 4-37 and 4-38).

▶ This nuclear/cytoplasmic asynchrony results in the formation of red cells known as megaloblasts.

▶ Megaloblasts have the following features:
  – Large cells
  – Immature, pale ("watery") nuclei with irregular chromatin clumps.
  – Cytoplasm is too hemoglobinized for the degree of nuclear maturation.

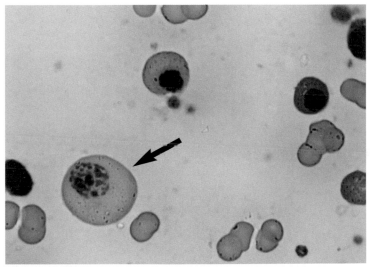

**Figure 4-37**
Feline blood. Nuclear maturation defect. Three NRBCs are present in the field. Two of the NRBCs have excessive polychromatophilic cytoplasm. The nucleus in one NRBC (arrow) is very large and has a reticulated chromatin pattern. This nucleus should be found in a cytoplasm that is dark blue with very little visible hemoglobin. The nucleus is maturing at a different rate than the cytoplasm indicating a severe defect in development. This cat had a severe anemia with a very high MCV but no increase in reticulocytes (100x).

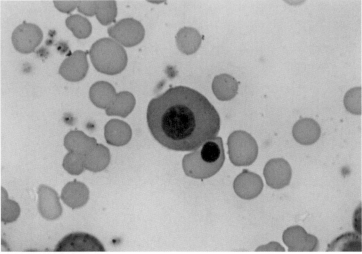

**Figure 4-38**
Feline blood. Nuclear maturation defect. Two NRBCs are located in the center of the field. The smaller NRBC appears normal. The larger cell has severe nuclear /cytoplasmic maturation defect. The nucleus in this cell is very immature for the degree of cytoplasmic development. This morphology is sometimes referred to as megaloblastic erythropoiesis. FeLV should be considered as a major cause of this abnormality (100x).

► The presence of megaloblasts in the marrow confirms the diagnosis.

► The nuclear defect is the result of abnormal/reduced DNA synthesis.

► The bone marrow is hypercellular; all cell lines are affected and left-shifted.

► While definitive diagnosis depends on bone marrow morphology, peripheral blood findings are suggestive:

– Mild pancytopenia is usual.

– The anemia generally presents with normocytic, normochromic to macrocytic, normochromic red cell indices.

– Occasional megaloblasts may be present on blood films.

– Occasional giant fully hemoglobinized red cells are present.

– Occasional red cells containing bizarre and/or multiple nuclear fragments may also be observed.

► Nuclear maturation defect anemias are far more common in cats than dogs.

► Nuclear maturation defect anemias are most commonly associated with FeLV infection in cats.

► Folic acid deficiency is also a cause.

► Chemotherapy can cause interference with DNA synthesis and nuclear development (methotrexate) resulting in megaloblastic change.

► Toy Poodles sometimes have megaloblastic red cells in the peripheral blood. In this breed, these findings are normal.

## Maturation Defect Anemias: Cytoplasmic Defect

► The principal defect in these anemias is failure to form hemoglobin; nuclear maturation of red cell precursors is normal.

► The result is a hypercellular red cell bone marrow with a build-up of small metarubricytes (Figure 4-39).

  – Red cell precursors continue to divide, getting smaller and smaller, because they never acquire a full complement of hemoglobin.

  – Normal reticulocytes are produced and released at a much reduced rate.

► Causes include:

  – Iron deficiency
  – Lead poisoning
  – B6 deficiency

► Iron deficiency and lead poisoning are by far the most important and are described in greater detail.

► Iron deficiency

  – The end stage of blood loss anemia.

  – Blood films reveal small red cells with an increased area of central pallor (microcytic, hypochromic).

  – Increased red cell fragility results in marked poikilocytosis and red cell fragmentation.

  – Some polychromasia may be observed but it is inadequate to return the red cell mass to normal.

► Lead poisoning

  – A true cytoplasmic maturation defect anemia; lead interferes with hemoglobin synthesis at several points.

  – Lead also causes marrow stromal damage which results in release of nucleated red cells into circulation.

  – The resultant peripheral blood findings are those of normocytic, normochromic, nonregenerative anemia with large numbers of nucleated red cells.

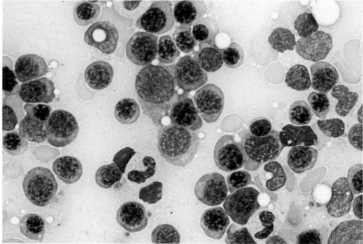

**Figure 4-39**
Canine bone marrow. Chronic hemorrhage. A marked increase in the late members of the erythroid series is present. Erythroid maturation is active up to the rubricyte and metarubricyte stages. Marrow iron stores are decreased due to chronic blood loss. These changes are consistent with iron deficiency anemia in the early stages (40x).

- ◆ Large numbers of nucleated red cells in the absence of an even greater number of polychromatophils is termed an inappropriate nucleated red cell response.
- – Inappropriate nucleated red cell responses of greater than 10 NRBC/100 WBC should cause the clinician to investigate the possibility of lead poisoning in dogs and FeLV infection in cats!.

## Hypoproliferative Non-regenerative Anemias (Erythroid Marrow Hypoplasia)

These anemias fall into three classes:

- ► Hypoproliferative anemia with granulocytic hyperplasia.
- ► Hypoproliferative anemia with selective erythroid hypoplasia.
- ► Hypoproliferative anemia with generalized marrow hypoplasia.

### Hypoproliferative Anemia with Granulocytic Hyperplasia

- ► This is the anemia of inflammatory disease (Figure 4-40).
- ► The anemia of inflammatory disease is the most common form of anemia in domestic animals and occurs with acute or chronic inflammation.
- ► Features include:

- Normocytic, normochromic anemia
- Anemia is mildly to moderately severe (hematocrits range from 20-35%).
- There is an inflammatory leukogram.
- Marrow smears are characterized by erythroid hypoplasia, granulocytic hyperplasia, increased marrow iron in marrow macrophages, and often increased numbers of plasma cells.

▶ This anemia can be associated with infections, neoplastic processes, and immune disorders.

## Anemias with Selective Erythroid Hypoplasia

▶ Peripheral blood findings include:
- Mild to severe normocytic normochromic anemias
- Normal white cell and platelet counts

▶ There are three major mechanisms involved in the genesis of selective erythroid hypoplasia.
- Reduced erythropoietin production (renal disease: Figure 4-41)
- Reduced oxygen demand and utilization by peripheral tissues (reduced basal metabolic rate as in hypothyroidism)

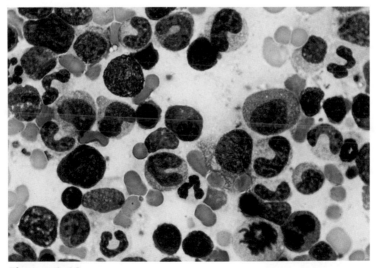

**Figure 4-40**
Canine bone marrow. Anemia of inflammation. The marrow is cellular in this dog (PCV = 33, inflammatory leukogram). The M:E ratio is increased due to granulocytic hyperplasia and erythroid hypoplasia. Plasma cells and iron stores are increased. These findings are consistent with the anemia of inflammation (40x).

– Selective destruction of red cell precursors by toxic or immune-mediated mechanisms. A complete history which includes enumeration of possible drug or chemical exposure is extremely important.

▶ Bone marrow evaluation is required for confirmation. Features include:
– Normal granulocyte and platelet production
– Rare red cell precursors
– Increased marrow iron
– Possible erythrophagocytosis by marrow macrophages

## Anemias with Generalized Marrow Hypoplasia
## (also known as aplastic anemias)

▶ Peripheral blood features include:
– Severe anemia
– Severe leukopenia
– Variable platelet counts, often severe thrombocytopenia

▶ Etiologic mechanisms fall into two major categories:
– Toxic or immune-mediated destruction of precursors in all cell lines (Figure 4-42).
– Myelophthisic anemias (replacement of marrow space by abnormal cellular elements)

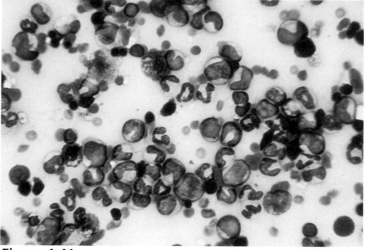

**Figure 4-41**
Feline bone marrow. Anemia of renal disease. Selective depression of erythropoiesis occurs in chronic renal disease due to diminished erythropoietin production. The M:E ratio is increased due to erythroid hypoplasia. Nearly all cells in the field are developing granulocytes (25x).

▶ Generalized marrow cytotoxicity can be caused by infectious agents, toxic chemicals, ionizing radiation, or immune destruction of marrow stem cells.
  – Infectious causes include FeLV and ehrlichiosis.
  – Toxic causes includes estrogen and chemotherapeutic agents such as Adriamycin.
  – Clinical presentation depends upon the severity of the various cell defects at diagnosis.
    ◆ If anemia is the most prevalent, then pale mucous membranes, lethargy, and anorexia are likely to be the presenting signs.
    ◆ With profound thrombocytopenia, bleeding will be the presenting problem.
    ◆ Where severe leukopenia is the primary problem, animals tend to present with serious infections.
  – Confirmation of diagnosis depends on marrow aspiration and core biopsy. Findings vary with the stage of the process.
▶ Myelophthisic anemias
  – May be caused by both neoplastic and non-neoplastic diseases.
  – The most common neoplastic causes are the hematopoietic and lymphoid neoplasms including granulocytic leukemia,

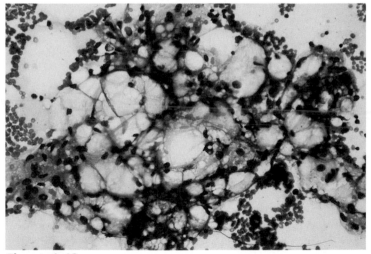

**Figure 4-42**
Feline bone marrow. Severe marrow hypoplasia. This cat presented with severe pancytopenia. Bone marrow is extremely hypocellular and contains adipose tissue and some connective tissue elements. Normal myeloid cells are rare. This cat had been treated with griseofulvin for a skin fungus. This drug can cause severe marrow hypoplasia in cats (25x).

lymphoid leukemias and lymphosarcoma, and erythremic myelosis (Figure 4-43).

– The principal non-neoplastic cause is myelofibrosis, the replacement of marrow spaces by connective tissue (Figure 4-44).

  ◆ Myelofibrosis may be the endpoint of previous severe marrow injury (as in the case of estrogen toxicity and ionizing radiation) or it may occur spontaneously.

– Peripheral blood features of myelofibrosis usually include severe nonregenerative anemia, severe leukopenia, and a variable platelet response.

  ◆ A striking morphologic feature of many cases of myelofibrosis is the presence of dacryocytes or tear-drop shaped erythrocytes on the blood film.

– Confirmation of the diagnosis depends on marrow core biopsy and histopathology with a demonstration of connective tissue filling marrow space.

# Polycythemia (Table 4-1)

Polycythemia is defined as increased circulating red cell mass.

Values for PCV, hemoglobin concentration, and RBC count are higher than reference ranges due to a relative or absolute increase in circulating RBCs.

Reference values for PCV, hemoglobin, and RBC count can vary with geographic location and breed.

▶ Animals at altitudes >6000 ft have higher values than those at sea level.

▶ Brachycephalic breeds have higher PCVs than normocephalic breeds.

Severity of clinical signs in polycythemic animals is proportional to the degree of RBC excess.

▶ At PCV values >65%, hyperviscosity, poor perfusion, and reduced oxygenation of tissues are present.

Polycythemias can be classified as relative, transient, or absolute.

## *Relative Polycythemia*

Relative polycythemia occurs when a decrease in plasma volume, usually due to dehydration, produces a relative increase in circulating RBCs.

▶ Clinical findings – Dehydration or shift of plasma $H_2O$ to interstitium or gastrointestinal lumen.

▶ Causes – Vomiting, diarrhea, diminished water intake, diuresis, hyperventilation, renal disease.

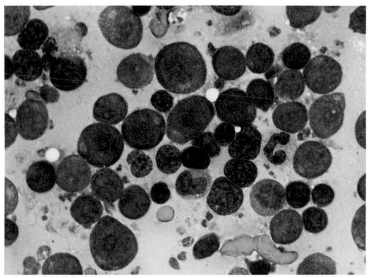

## Figure 4-43

Canine bone marrow. Myelophthisis. Normal myeloid cells have been replaced by a population of dark round blast cells. Two neutrophils are visible in the entire field. Closer examination of the cells confirmed a diagnosis of lymphoma (40x).

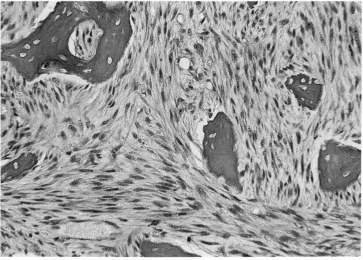

## Figure 4-44

Core biopsy of bone marrow. Myelofibrosis. The marrow spaces contain palisading layers of fibrous connective tissue instead of developing granulocytes and erythroid precursors. This dog was pancytopenic, and repeated attempts to aspirate bone marrow were unsuccessful (40x).

## TABLE 4-1  Laboratory Features of Polycythemias

|  | RELATIVE | ABSOLUTE | | |
|---|---|---|---|---|
|  |  | Primary | Secondary | Secondary |
| Mechanism | Dehydration | Myelopro-liferative | Hypoxemia | Excess EPO |
| PCV | Increased | Marked Inc >60% | Marked Inc >60% | Marked Inc >60% |
| Plasma protein concentration | Increased | Normal | Normal | Normal |
| Arterial $O_2$ saturation |  | Normal >90% | Decrease <<90% | Normal >90% |
| Plasma erythropoietin |  | Normal | Increased | Increased |
| Bone Marrow | Normal | ————Erythroid hyperplasia———— | | |
| Other | Prerenal azotemia | Inc WBC Inc Plat | | |

▶ Laboratory features: Moderate increase in PCV and total protein concentration in plasma. Prerenal azotemia may also be present.

## Transient Polycythemia

Transient polycythemia is caused by splenic contraction which injects concentrated RBC into circulation.

▶ Occurs in anxious or excitable dogs or cats and subsides within an hour.

▶ Large excitable breeds are prone to splenic contraction.

▶ Laboratory features: Increase in PCV with normal hydration and normal total protein concentration in plasma.

## Absolute Polycythemias

Absolute polycythemia is characterized by an absolute increase in the circulating RBCs as a result of increased marrow production.

▶ Classified as either primary, or secondary to increased production of EPO.

▶ Animals with absolute polycythemia have an expanded blood volume.

▶ Clinical findings – General lethargy, low exercise tolerance, behavioral change, brick red or cyanotic mucous membranes, sneezing, bilateral epistaxis, increased size and tortuosity of retinal and sublingual vessels, or cardiopulmonary impairment.

Primary absolute polycythemia (polycythemia rubra vera) is a rare myeloproliferative disorder characterized by the uncontrolled but orderly production of excessive numbers of mature RBCs.

▶ Clinical findings – In addition to above, variable degrees of splenomegaly, hepatomegaly, thrombosis, hemorrhage, and seizure activity.

▶ Hyperviscosity may result in thrombosis, infarction, or hemorrhage.

▶ Laboratory features: Marked increase in PCV (values of 65-75%) with erythroid hyperplasia in marrow. Clinical evidence of hypoxemia is not apparent. Erythropoietin levels are normal or reduced.

Secondary absolute polycythemia is caused by a physiologically appropriate release of EPO resulting from chronic hypoxemia.

▶ Clinical findings – Hypoxemia as a result of chronic pulmonary disease, cardiac disease or anomaly with right to left shunting, or hemoglobinopathy.

▶ Causes – Chronic pulmonary disease, cardiac disease, cardiac anomaly with right to left shunting, high altitude, brachycephalic breeds, methemoglobinemia, and impairment of renal blood supply.

▶ Laboratory features: Moderate to marked increase in PCV and marrow erythroid hyperplasia with decreased arterial $PO_2$ content. Erythropoietin levels are increased.

Secondary absolute polycythemia is also caused by an inappropriate and excessive production of EPO or an EPO-like substance in an animal with normal arterial oxygen saturation.

▶ Clinical findings – Signs associated with renal or hepatic neoplasia, space-occupying renal lesion, or endocrine disorder.

▶ Causes – Renal cyst or tumor, hydronephrosis, hyperadrenocorticism, hyperthyroidism, pheochromocytoma, nasal fibrosarcoma, hepatic neoplasia, hyperandrogenism

▶ Laboratory features: Moderate or marked increase in PCV with marrow erythroid hyperplasia and a normal arterial $PO_2$ content. Erythropoietin levels plasma are increased.

# 5

# Neutrophils

# OVERVIEW
## Origin

Neutrophils are produced in the bone marrow, released into blood, circulate briefly, and migrate into tissue spaces or on to epithelial surfaces such as those in the respiratory, digestive, or urogenital tracts.

Production is continuous in order to provide for the continual demand for neutrophils in the tissues and maintain the circulating pool in the blood.

Transit time for generation of neutrophils in marrow is approximately 4-6 days and the marrow maintains a five day supply of mature neutrophils in storage.

Injury or bacterial invasion of tissue results in the production and release of colony-stimulating factors (CSFs) that govern the proliferation and maturation of immature neutrophils in the marrow.

Granulopoiesis is a continuum of cell division, differentiation, and maturation (Figure 5-1).
▶ Stem cells differentiate into myeloblasts which are the earliest recognizable cell in the granulocytic series.
▶ Division and differentiation of myeloblasts result in sequential generations of progranulocytes and myelocytes.
▶ Subsequent generations consist of metamyelocytes, bands, and segmented neutrophils which are postmitotic cells that undergo nuclear and cytoplasmic changes to become capable of phagocytosis and microbicidal activity.

Neutrophils circulate for about 10 hours in blood and are compartmentalized into a circulating neutrophil pool and a marginal neutrophil pool.
▶ Neutrophils in the circulating neutrophil pool circulate with other blood cells and are measured in the CBC.
▶ The marginal neutrophil pool consists of neutrophils that adhere intermittently to endothelium especially in small veins and capillaries. These cells are not counted in the CBC.
▶ In dogs the ratio of neutrophils in the circulating to marginal pools is 1:1. For cats, the ratio is 1:3.

Migration of neutrophils into tissues occurs randomly and is unidirectional.
▶ Neutrophils survive for 1-4 days in tissues and undergo programmed cell death or apoptosis.

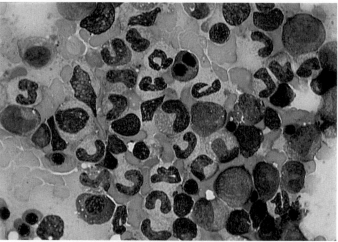

**Figure 5-1**
Normal granulopoiesis in canine bone marrow. The majority of cells are developing granulocytes. Segmented neutrophils and bands predominate with fewer numbers of metamyelocytes, myelocytes, progranulocytes (60x).

▶ Neutrophils are also destroyed in spleen, liver, and bone marrow by resident macrophages.

Factors that influence the numbers of circulating neutrophils include the relative rates of:

▶ Bone marrow production and release.

▶ Exchange between circulating neutrophil pool and marginal neutrophil pool.

▶ Migration into tissue.

# Function

Neutrophils serve as the primary defense against invasion of tissues by microorganisms. Neutrophils kill bacteria and can also damage or participate in the destruction of mycotic agents, algae, and viruses.

Neutrophils accumulate at sites of inflammation or bacterial infection by a process of directional migration or chemotaxis.

▶ Cellular and molecular mediators of inflammation generate chemotactic substances, stimulate marrow release, and promote margination and adhesion of neutrophils to vascular endothelium at sites of inflammation.

▶ Neutrophils leave the blood stream and enter the tissues by transmigration between endothelial cells.

At the site of inflammation, neutrophils are capable of phagocytosis and microbicidal activity. Fusion of lysosomal granules with the phagocytic vesicle releases lytic enzymes and chemicals capable of killing bacteria.

# QUANTITY

Changes in the rates of marrow production and release, the exchange between marginal neutrophil pool and circulating neutrophil pool, and/or the rate of tissue migration directly influence the number of neutrophils measured in a CBC.

WBCs and neutrophils counted electronically via impedance can be falsely increased by large platelets, platelet clumps, and Heinz bodies. Leukocyte clumping causes a false decrease in WBC count.

## Neutropenia

A decrease in the absolute number of neutrophils.

In dogs and cats, neutropenia occurs when the absolute count is less than 3000-4000/$\mu$l.

Neutropenia is the most frequent cause of leukopenia.

Mechanisms of neutropenia include (Figure 5-4):
- ▶ Acute demand or consumption in tissues
- ▶ Decreased marrow production
- ▶ Ineffective granulopoiesis (dysgranulopoiesis)
- ▶ Increased margination from the circulating neutrophil pool to the marginal neutrophil pool

### Neutropenia Due to Acute Tissue Demand
- ▶ Neutrophils can rapidly sequester in a well-vascularized tissue that becomes acutely inflamed or septic (Figure 5-2).
- ▶ Neutropenia results when the rate of migration into tissue exceeds the capacity of the marrow storage pool of neutrophils.
  - – The inflammatory process is so severe and acute that there is insufficient time for granulopoiesis to replenish the supply of mature neutrophils.
  - – Bands and some metamyelocytes are released from the marrow causing a severe left shift.
- ▶ Toxic change often will be evident in neutrophils in blood and in precursors in marrow.

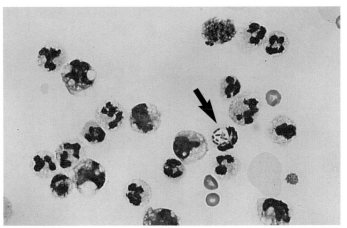

**Figure 5-2**
Neutrophilic exudate from a dog with bacterial peritonitis. The majority
of cells are degenerate neutrophils. Rod-shaped bacteria (arrow) have
been phagocytosed by a neutrophil (60x).

▶ Neutropenia with a severe left shift and toxic neutrophils is seen
in conditions such as acute peritonitis, ruptured GI viscus, acute
metritis, gangrenous mastitis, and acute cellulitis.

▶ A poor or guarded prognosis is indicated because of the extent
and severity of inflammation necessary to produce this neutrophil
response. (See Case 11 and Case 13.)

## Neutropenia Due to Decreased Marrow Production

▶ Severe toxic insults to marrow can result in decreased marrow
production of neutrophils.

▶ The bone marrow in these animals is usually hypocellular with a
severe reduction in granulocytic, erythroid and megakaryocytic precursors (Figure 5-3). On occasion, the marrow is very cellular due to
extensive replacement by neoplastic cells (myelophthisis).

▶ Potential causes include: adverse drug reactions, exposure to toxic
chemicals and plants, infectious agents, myelophthisis, and suspected
immune-mediated marrow destruction.

▶ Drugs that have been incriminated include: estrogen, phenylbutazone, trimethoprim-sulfadiazine, chloramphenicol, griseofulvin,
and several chemotherapeutic agents.

▶ Infectious agents include: parvovirus, panleukopenia virus, feline
leukemia virus, *Ehrlichia*.

▶ Production of RBCs and platelets can also be affected resulting in
concurrent nonregenerative anemia and thrombocytopenia. (See Case 10)

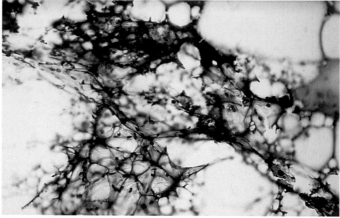

**Figure 5-3**
Severe marrow hypoplasia in a dog resulting in neutropenia, anemia, and thrombocytopenia. The hematopoietic cells are markedly reduced and have been replaced by fat tissue (40x).

## *Neutropenia Due to Ineffective Granulopoiesis (dysgranulopoiesis)*

▶ Neutropenia can occur because of arrested development or a reduction in marrow release in spite of adequate numbers of granulocytic progenitor cells in marrow.

▶ The bone marrow in these animals is cellular with adequate or increased numbers of granulocytic precursors.

▶ Diseases associated with this neutrophil response include: myelodysplasia, acute myeloid leukemia, and infections caused by feline leukemia or feline immunodeficiency virus.

## *Neutropenia Due to Increased Margination*

▶ A sudden shift in neutrophils from the circulating neutrophil pool to the marginal neutrophil pool can cause a transient acute neutropenia.

▶ Causes include:
– Anaphylaxis
– Endotoxemia

▶ Neutropenia is an early, transient event and may disappear before the animal is presented for medical treatment. (Figure 5-4)

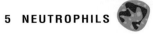

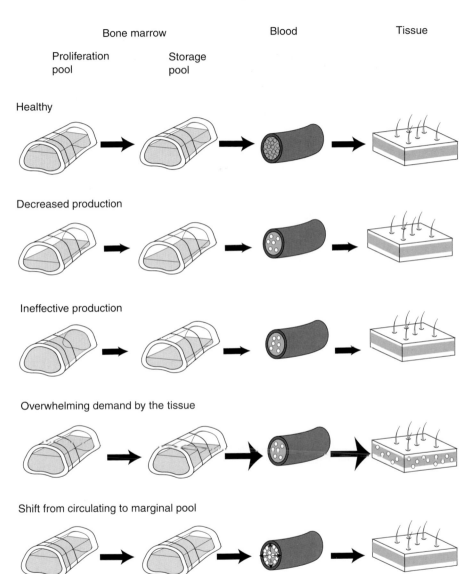

## Figure 5-4

Mechanisms of neutropenia. Changes in the production, distribution, release, and circulation are indicated in bone marrow and blood. Relative size of arrows indicates changes in rate of release from blood and bone marrow and the rate of migration into tissue. Modified from Schalm's Veterinary Hematology.

# Neutrophilia

Neutrophilia is defined as an increase in the absolute numbers of circulating neutrophils. In adult dogs and cats, neutrophil counts exceed 12,000-13,000/µl. Neutrophilia is the most frequent cause of leukocytosis. Causes of neutrophilia include (Figure 5-5):

► Physiologic or epinephrine-induced
► Corticosteroid- or stress-induced
► Acute inflammation
► Chronic inflammation with marked neutrophilia
► Chronic inflammation with new steady state
► Hemorrhage or hemolysis
► Granulocytic leukemia
► Inherited granulocyte defects

## Physiologic Neutrophilia

► Epinephrine release causes a transient (1 hour) mature neutrophilia by shifting neutrophils from the marginal neutrophil pool to the circulating neutrophil pool.
► Epinephrine release is caused by fear, excitement, vigorous exercise, and seizure activity.
► In cats, a marked lymphocytosis (6000 to 20,000/µl) can occur concurrently or be the prevalent finding. (See Case 1.)

## Corticosteroid or Stress-Induced Neutrophilia

► Increased circulating levels of glucocorticoids cause increased release of mature neutrophils into the circulating neutrophils and decreased migration of neutrophils into tissue.
► The response can occur after endogenous secretion or exogenous administration of corticosteroids. Common causes of endogenous release include pain, traumatic injury, boarding, transport, or other painful conditions.
► Following exogenous administration, leukocytosis (17,000-35,000/µl) and neutrophilia occur within 4-8 hours and return to normal 1-3 days after treatment. (See Case 2.)

## Neutrophilia of Acute Inflammation

► Inflammation, sepsis, necrosis, or immune-mediated disease cause increased tissue demand and increased marrow release of segmented and band neutrophils.

► Leukocytosis (15,000-30,000/μl) characterized by neutrophilia with left shift and variable monocytosis is the usual response. Toxic neutrophils may be observed.

► Lymphopenia and eosinopenia, reflections of stress and elevated circulating glucocorticoids, are also common.

► Surgical removal or drainage of septic focus may transiently increase the magnitude of the neutrophilia. (See Case 11.)

## Neutrophilia of Chronic Inflammation

► Some chronic suppurative lesions (eg, pyometra, abscesses, pyothorax, pyoderma) and some neoplasms can cause marrow granulocytic hyperplasia that results in severe leukocytosis (50,000-120,000).

► Laboratory features include neutrophilia with a left shift, variable numbers of toxic neutrophils, monocytosis, and often hyperglobulinemia.

► The anemia of inflammation (mild to moderate nonregenerative anemia) is usually present.

► The term "leukemoid response" is used to describe such inflammatory neutrophilias with WBC counts >100,000/μl. (See Case 9.)

## Chronic Inflammation with New Steady State

► A second form of chronic inflammation is seen where a new steady state has been reached between marrow production and release of granulocytes and tissue demand.

► Total white cell counts are normal or only slightly elevated.

► Neutrophil counts are high normal or only slightly elevated and there is minimal to no left shift.

► Lymphocyte numbers tend to be in the reference range.

► The most consistent leukogram abnormality is monocytosis.

► The anemia of inflammatory disease and hyperglobulinemia are often present. (See Case 6.)

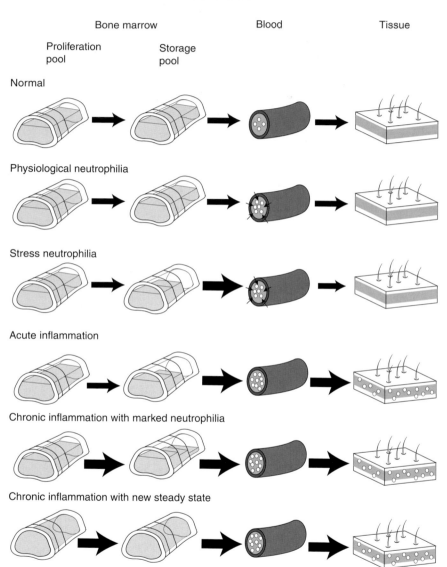

Neutrophilia

Bone marrow

Proliferation pool

Storage pool

Blood

Tissue

Normal

Physiological neutrophilia

Stress neutrophilia

Acute inflammation

Chronic inflammation with marked neutrophilia

Chronic inflammation with new steady state

## Figure 5-5

Mechanisms of neutrophilia changes in production, distribution, release and circulation are indicated in bone marrow and blood. Relative size of arrows indicates changes in rate of release from blood and bone marrow and the rate of migration into tissue.

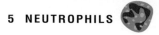

### Hemolytic or Hemorrhagic Anemias
▶ Neutrophilias with left shift frequently occur in animals with immune-mediated hemolytic anemia. Leukocytosis can be marked (>50,000/μl).

▶ Mature neutrophilia occurs 3 hours following acute hemorrhage. (See Case 8.)

### Chronic Granulocytic Leukemia
▶ Usually presents with marked neutrophilic leukocytosis (>80,000/μl).

▶ Left shift is present and may be disordered with evidence of a maturation arrest. Very young neutrophil precursors (promyelocytes and myeloblasts) may be seen.

▶ Thrombocytopenia and/or nonregenerative anemia are observed in varying degrees.

▶ Hepatomegaly and/or splenomegaly may be present due to neoplastic infiltration.

▶ This condition must be differentiated from the neutrophilia of chronic inflammation. (See Case 18.)

### Inherited Neutrophil Disorders
▶ Consider only when other causes can be eliminated.

▶ B$_2$ integrin deficiency has been recognized in Irish Setters and results in decreased neutrophil adhesion to endothelium, diminished chemotaxis, and decreased bactericidal activity. These dogs have persistent neutrophilia and recurrent infections.

▶ Cyclic hematopoiesis or grey colic syndrome is characterized by cyclic fluctuations in neutrophils, monocytes, eosinophils, platelets, and reticulocytes at 11-13 day intervals. Neutrophil changes are most pronounced with neutrophilia following 2 to 4 day neutropenic episodes.

# MORPHOLOGY
## Normal

Normal circulating neutrophils have the following features (Figures 5-6 and 5-7):
▶ Size – 12-15 μ in diameter or 2-2.5 times the diameter of a RBC.

▶ Nucleus – lobulated or partially segmented with dense, dark purple chromatin.

► Cytoplasm – pale pink or light blue, finely granular, smooth

Most of the circulating neutrophils (95-100%) in normal animals are segmented forms. Very few are band neutrophils.

Variation in normal morphology (Figures 5-8 and 5-9)

► Prolonged exposure to EDTA prior to preparing the blood film can produce discrete, clear, cytoplasmic vacuoles in the cytoplasm.

► Normal neutrophils have two to four nuclear lobes.

► Five or more lobes indicate hypersegmentation, an aging change, which occurs with prolonged exposure to EDTA, glucocorticoid therapy, hyperadrenocorticism, or neutrophilias associated with chronic infections.

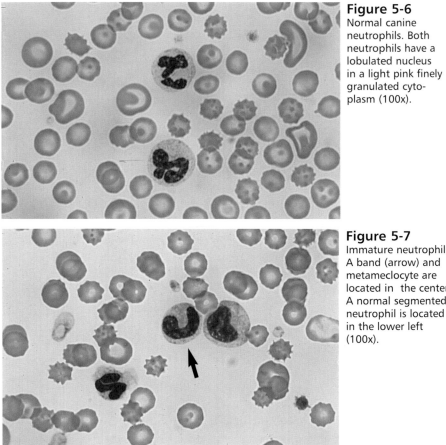

**Figure 5-6**
Normal canine neutrophils. Both neutrophils have a lobulated nucleus in a light pink finely granulated cytoplasm (100x).

**Figure 5-7**
Immature neutrophils. A band (arrow) and metameclocyte are located in the center. A normal segmented neutrophil is located in the lower left (100x).

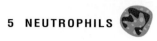

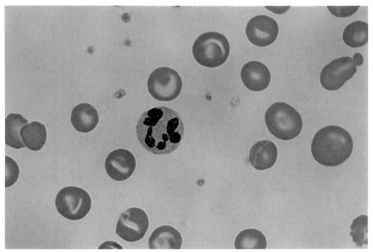

### Figure 5-8
Hypersegmented neutrophil. Dog and cat neutrophils may have up to five nuclear lobes. This neutrophil has 8 nuclear lobes and is evidence of prolonged lifespan (100x).

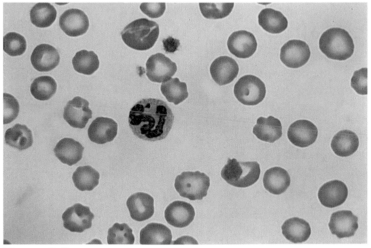

### Figure 5-9
Canine neutrophil with Barr body. The small tennis racket shaped appendage on the neutrophil nucleus is a Barr body, or sex lobe, indicating that the dog is a female. This can be a useful morphologic feature in dogs and cats if there is a question of gender or patient identity (100x).

# In Disease

Toxic neutrophils (Figures 5-10A, 5-10B, and 5-10C)
- ▶ Morphologic changes are apparent in neutrophils of dogs and cats with severe inflammatory disease or toxemia.
- ▶ The severity of the morphologic changes is proportional to the intensity of the inflammatory or toxemic disease.
- ▶ Morphologic features of toxic neutrophils:
  - – Diffuse cytoplasmic basophilia – color of the cytoplasm becomes blue-grey.
  - – Foamy vacuolation of the cytoplasm – irregular clearing in the cytoplasm produces vacuolation.
  - – Dohle bodies – one or more, irregular, basophilic cytoplasmic inclusions.
  - – Abnormal nuclear shapes – irregular lobulation or ring shaped nuclei.
- ▶ Toxic change is scored as mild, moderate, or severe  on a scale of 1+ to 3+.

Infectious agents (Figures 5-11 and 5-12)
- ▶ Organisms that can be found in neutrophil cytoplasms include *Ehrlichia*, *Hepatozoon*, and *Histoplasma*.
- ▶ Canine distemper inclusions are seen occasionally in neutrophil and lymphocyte cytoplasms.

Neutrophil changes with inherited disorders
- ▶ Lysosomal Storage Disease – Cats and dogs with mucopolysacharidoses, gangliosidosis have fine, purple cytoplasmic granules in neutrophils (Figure 5-13).
- ▶ Chediak-Higashi Syndrome – small, round pink granules are present in neutrophil cytoplasm.
- ▶ Pelger Huet Anomaly (Figure 5-14)
  - – Occasionally seen in dogs.
  - – Neutrophil and eosinophil nuclei are hyposegmented but have dark, condensed mature chromatin patterns.
  - – Neutrophils and eosinophils are functionally normal so the condition is not clinically significant.
  - – Must be differentiated from a true left shift.
  - – Also occurs in rabbits where the anomaly occurs in association with other fatal heritable abnormalities.

## Figure 5-10

Toxic neutrophils. With
severe inflammation or toxemia, neutrophils develop
morphologic changes that
include cytoplasmic baso-
philia, cytoplasmic vacuolation, Dohle bodies, cytoplasmic granulation, and bizarre
nuclear configuration. All
three pictures demonstrate
cytoplasmic basophilia.
Neutrophils in **A** and **B** have
Dohle bodies (arrows). **C**
shows feline blood with the
neutrophils having a
basophilic granular cyto-
plasm and a bizarre circular
nucleus.

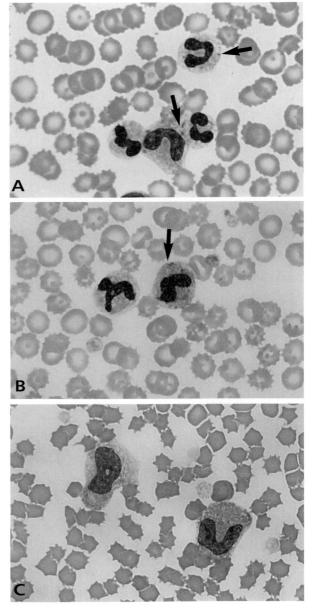

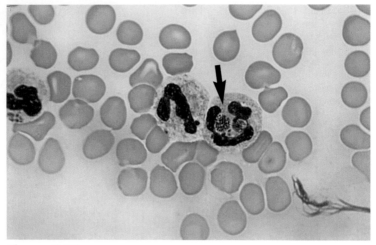

**Figure 5-11**
Canine Ehrlichia: Round, granular, basophilic inclusion in neutrophil cytoplasm (arrow) is an *Ehrlichia* morula (100x).

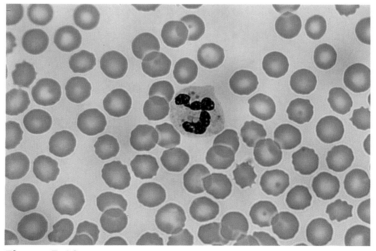

**Figure 5-12**
Canine distemper inclusion bodies. Pale light pink, round cytoplasmic
droplets in the neutrophil are canine distemper viral inclusions (100x).

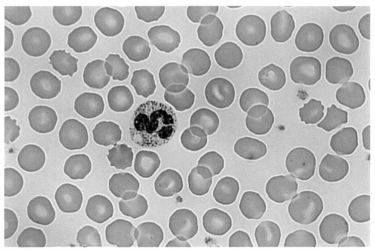

**Figure 5-13**
Neutrophil from a dog with lysosomal storage disease. Numerous small basophilic granules are noted in the cytoplasm of a segmented neutrophil of a dog with gangliosidosis. Neutrophils from cats with mucopolysaccaridosis have a similar appearance (100x).

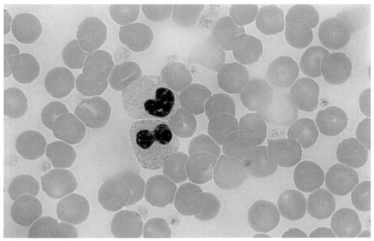

**Figure 5-14**
Canine blood, Pelger Huet anomaly. This inherited disorder causes hyposegmentation of neutrophil and eosinophil nuclei, giving the appearance of a persistent left shift. However, the neutrophils do not have toxic change and the nuclear chromatin is very dark and condensed indicating maturity (100x).

# 6
# Eosinophils

# OVERVIEW
## Origin

Eosinophils are produced in the bone marrow in a process similar to neutrophil production.

Eosinophils are recognizable at the myelocytes stage with the appearance of eosinophil specific granules.

IL-5 produced by sensitized T lymphocytes is the major cytokine that stimulates eosinophil production.

Marrow generation time and storage of eosinophils are similar to neutrophils.

## Function

Eosinophils participate as a major component of systemic hypersensitivity reactions.
> ▶ When parasite antigens or allergens bind to specific IgE on mast cells, the mast cells degranulate and release histamine which attracts eosinophils.

Eosinophils play a major role in killing flukes and nematodes that have IgG or complement bound to their surface.

Eosinophils have limited phagocytic and bactericidal activity and may play a role in destroying neoplastic cells.

# QUANTITY

Eosinophil numbers in circulation reflect a balance of marrow production and demand or consumption in tissue.
> ▶ A variety of diseases are characterized by a marked eosinophilic inflammatory cell response in tissue. These diseases may or may not be accompanied by an eosinophilia in blood.

There is considerable geographic variation in reference ranges for eosinophils.
> ▶ Ranges are higher in the south and east coastal regions of North America than for the northern and central plains areas.
> ▶ It is important to use species reference ranges generated from animals resident in the region.

# Eosinopenia

Eosinopenia is defined as a reduction in circulating eosinophils.
- In most laboratories, the lower limit for absolute number of eosinophils is zero (0) or a very small number. Therefore, eosinopenia is best detected in sequential CBCs.

Endogenous secretion or administration of glucocorticoids results in eosinopenia by reducing marrow release and increasing eosinophil sequestration and apoptosis in tissue.

Because eosinophils are reduced with increased glucocorticoids levels, causes of eosinophilia should be considered in a stressed animal with a normal eosinophil count.

# Eosinophilia

Eosinophilia is defined as an increase in absolute eosinophil count.

Causes of eosinophilia include:
- Allergy – IgE-mediated hypersensitivity reactions are likely causes especially when the animal experiences re-exposure to the inciting allergen.
- Parasites – Flukes, nematodes, or ectoparasites that have significant tissue migration or tissue contact phase.
- Granulomatous inflammation – Chronic granulomatous disease causes by fungi or foreign bodies.
- Neoplasms – Mast cell tumors and less frequently lymphomas can evoke an eosinophilia. A neoplasm that is heavily infiltrated with eosinophils may have a more favorable prognosis that one that is free of eosinophils.
- Hypereosinophilic syndrome – Difficult to differentiate from eosinophilic leukemia. Usually considered after other causes are eliminated.
- Eosinophilic leukemia – Extremely rare myeloproliferative neoplasm in cats. Eosinophilia is present with immature forms in blood. Eosinophil infiltrates are also seen in liver, spleen, and lymph nodes.

Allergic, parasitic, or inflammatory diseases that occur in the skin, gastrointestinal tract, lung, or female genital tract are most likely to produce eosinophilia.

# MORPHOLOGY

There are marked species differences in eosinophil morphology.

Canine eosinophils
- ▶ Size – 12-20 $\mu$ in diameter or similar or slightly larger than a neutrophil.
- ▶ Nucleus – lobulated or partially segmented with dense, dark purple chromatin.
- ▶ Cytoplasm – orange-red granules that are round and vary in size and number (Figures 6-1A and 6-1B. On occasion, canine eosinophil may contain one large solitary round granule that is similar in size and color to a RBC (Figure 6-1C).

Feline eosinophils (Figures 6-2A, 6-2B, and 6-3)
- ▶ Size – 12-20 $\mu$ in diameter or, similar or slightly larger than a neutrophil.
- ▶ Nucleus – lobulated or segmented with dark purple chromatin.
- ▶ Cytoplasm – numerous, light pink rod-shaped granules.

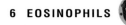

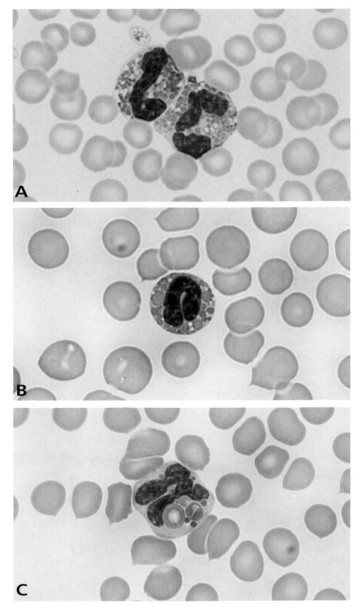

## Figure 6-1

Canine eosinophils. Granules in canine eosinophils are round and can vary in size and number. **A.** Granules are numerous, round, and small. **B.** A few granules are present and size variation is more pronounced. **C.** This eosinophil contains a few large round granules. In this cell, the granules appear similar in size and color to the surrounding RBCs (100x).

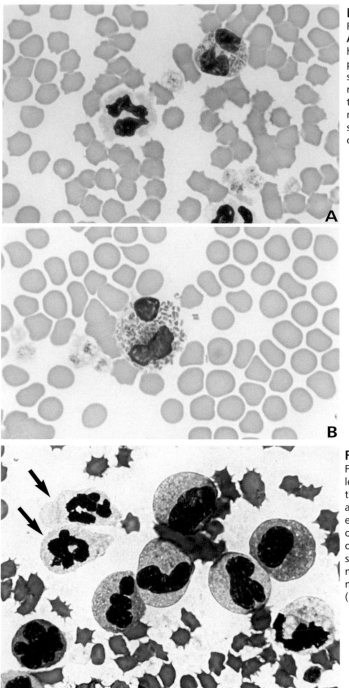

**Figure 6-2**
Feline eosinophils.
**A.** Eosinophil (top) has granules that are pale pink and rod-shaped. **B.** The cell membrane has ruptured in smear preparation and the rod-shaped granules are clearly visible (100x).

A

B

**Figure 6-3**
Feline eosinophilic leukemia. Two neutrophils (arrows) are adjacent to several eosinophils at various stages of development that include segmented, band, metamyelocyte, and myelocyte forms (100x).

# 7

# Basophils

# OVERVIEW
## Origin

Basophils are produced in the bone marrow and share a common progenitor cell with tissue mast cells. Basophils do not develop into mast cells, but the two cell types have similar functions.

Immature basophils can be recognized at the myelocytes stage by their characteristic secondary granules.

Maturation through the metamyelocyte, band, and segmented stages in marrow take about 2.5 days.

Basophils circulate for a few hours in blood and migrate into tissues where they may reside for several weeks.

## Function

Basophil granules contain histamine and heparin.

▶ Histamine release from basophils and mast cells plays a significant role in immediate hypersensitivity reactions such as occurs in urticaria, anaphylaxis, and acute allergy.

▶ Heparin inhibits coagulation, which has an important role in inflammation.

▶ Activated basophils synthesize several cytokines that initiate or modulate the inflammatory response.

# QUANTITY

Basophils comprise a very low percentage of the circulating leukocyte population. In most dogs and cats, basophils will rarely be observed in a manual leukocyte differential count.

## Basopenia

Since basophils are seen rarely in peripheral blood, it is difficult to assess basopenia. Endogenous or exogenous glucocorticoids cause a reduction in circulating basophils.

## Basophilia

Causes of basophilia should be considered in a dog or cat with a persistent basophil count of 200-300/$\mu$l. Basophilia often occurs concurrently with eosinophilia.

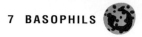

Causes of basophilia include:
- ▶ Allergy and hypersensitivity reaction
- ▶ Parasites – Nematodes, flukes, or ectoparasites that have a significant tissue migration or tissue contact phase. Dirofilaria, tick infestation, or flea allergy are frequent causes.
- ▶ Hyperlipemia – Metabolic or endocrine disorders associated with lipemia may be accompanied by basophilia.
- ▶ Basophilic leukemia – Extremely rare myeloproliferative neoplasm

## MORPHOLOGY

There are marked species differences in basophil morphology.

Canine basophil
- ▶ Size – 12-20 μ in diameter or, similar or slightly larger than a neutrophil.
- ▶ Nucleus – segmented lobulated nucleus (Figure 7-1A)
- ▶ Cytoplasm – light purple or grey with a few discrete dark granules (Figure 7-1B). Granules may be very sparse or absent in some cells.

Feline basophil
- ▶ Size – 12-20 μ in diameter, or slightly larger than a neutrophil.
- ▶ Nucleus – segmented lobulated nucleus with light smooth chromatin very similar to the nucleus in a monocyte.
- ▶ Cytoplasm – numerous round, lavender granules (Figures 7-2A, 7-2B).

Mast Cells
- ▶ Size – similar to basophils in cat and dog.
- ▶ Nucleus – round to oval, central or eccentric location in cytoplasm.
- ▶ Cytoplasm – numerous small round, dark purple granules that may partially obscure the nucleus (Figures 7-3 and 7-4).

Mast cells are rarely seen in peripheral blood.

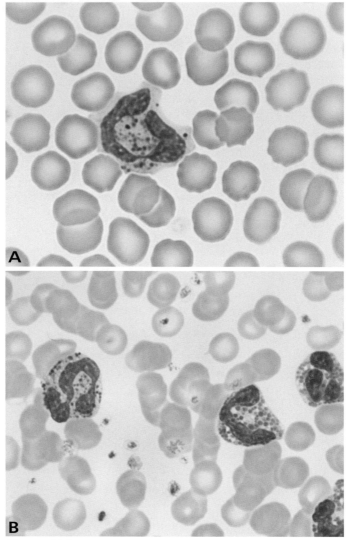

**Figure 7-1**
Canine basophils. **A.** Lobulated nucleus is present in a grey cytoplasm with a few basophilic granules. **B.** The basophil (left) has darker cytoplasmic granules compared with the orange pink granules in the eosinophils (100x).

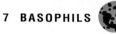

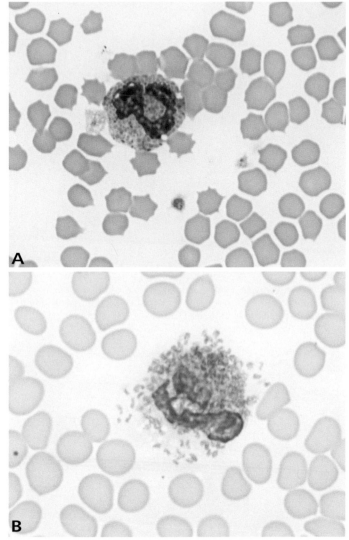

## Figure 7-2

Feline basophil. **A.** Numerous round lavender granules surround a lobulated nucleus. Feline basophils can be easily confused with monocytes. **B.** The cell membrane has ruptured in smear preparation and the lavender cytoplasmic granules are clearly visible (100x).

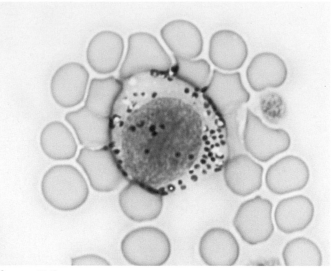

**Figure 7-3**
Mast cell leukemia in a cat. Mast cells have a round nucleus with a moderate amount of cytoplasm. This mast cell contains only a few basophilic cytoplasmic granules (100x).

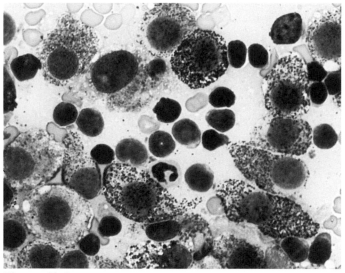

**Figure 7-4**
Fine needle aspirate of a lymph node. Metastasis of a cutaneous mast cell tumor to a regional lymph node. Numerous well-granulated mast cells are present with a few small lymphocytes (60x).

# 8

# Monocytes

# OVERVIEW
## Origin
Monocytes originate in the bone marrow.

▶ Unlike granulocytes, they are released into the peripheral blood as immature cells and are transported to the tissues where they can differentiate into macrophages, epithelioid cells, or multinucleated inflammatory giant cells.

▶ The circulating monocyte is comparable in degree of differentiation to the neutrophilic myelocytes found in the bone marrow.

There is no bone marrow storage pool for monocytes.

▶ Monocytes and their precursors (monoblast, promonocyte) are present in low numbers and may be difficult to recognize.

▶ Increased monocyte production is reflected by increased numbers of circulating monocytes.

## Function

The monocyte/macrophage continuum represents the second major branch of the circulating phagocyte system (neutrophils being the first). Specific macrophage functions include:

▶ Phagocytosis

▶ Regulation of the inflammatory response via release of inflammatory mediators (chemotactic factors, prostaglandins, complement fragments, etc.)

▶ Antigen processing for presentation to lymphocytes; involved in the initiation of the immune response

▶ Participation in the regulation of body iron stores

# QUANTITY

Monocytopenia – reduced numbers of circulating monocytes – is not a recognized clinical entity.

Monocytosis is defined as increased numbers of circulating monocytes.

Monocytosis indicates:

▶ The presence of inflammation

▶ Demand for phagocytosis

▶ Tissue necrosis

Mild monocytosis can be associated with a "stress response" induced by high circulating glucocorticoids. This response is nonspecific.

# MORPHOLOGY
## Normal
Monocyte morphology is similar for dogs and cats.

Normal circulating monocytes have the following features.

► Size – 15-20 m

► Nucleus – irregular shape, lacy reticulated chromatin pattern(Figures 8-1A and 8-1B)

► Cytoplasm – abundant, grey to blue-grey

Variations in normal morphology can be related to sample handling.

► Monocytes in films made from fresh non-coagulated blood usually are round and contain no cytoplasmic vacuoles

► Monocytes in films made from EDTA-treated blood may have irregular cell margins with pseudopodia. They often contain cytoplasmic vacuoles.

## In Disease

Circulating monocytes can differentiate into macrophages if there is demand for phagocytosis in the blood.

► Nuclei become round to oval (Figure 8-2).

► Cytoplasm becomes more abundant.

► Vacuoles become more prominent and may contain phagocytized material of diagnostic significance (Figure 8-3):

– Red blood cells in cases of immune-mediated hemolytic anemia.

– Yeasts in diseases such as systemic histoplasmosis.

– Protozoal forms in diseases such as leishmaniasis.

Whenever monocytosis is marked, buffy coat smears should be made to concentrate monocytes to facilitate their evaluation for phagocytized material.

► Use freshly collected blood and make buffy coat smears promptly.

► If blood is allowed to stand in EDTA, some monocytes differentiate into macrophages and phagocytize damaged red cells and even other leukocytes. Such a finding is **not** indicative of disease.

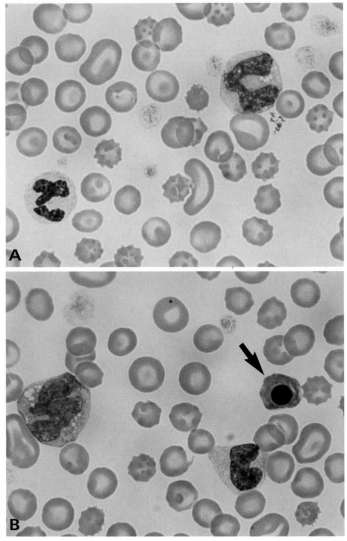

## Figure 8-1

Canine monocytes. Monocytes are slightly larger than a neutrophil and have a blue-grey cytoplasm, lobulated nucleus, and a lacy chromatin pattern. **A.** A segemented neutrophil (left) and a monocyte (right). **B.** The monocyte (left) contains a few round clear cytoplasmic vacuoles. A band neutrophil and an NRBC (arrow) are on the right (100x).

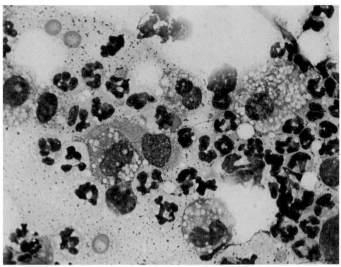

**Figure 8-2**
Fine needle aspirate of a granulomatous skin lesion. Neutrophils are adjacent to large macrophages that have abundant vacuolated cytoplasm and round to oval nuclei. Macrophages are derived from blood monocytes (100x).

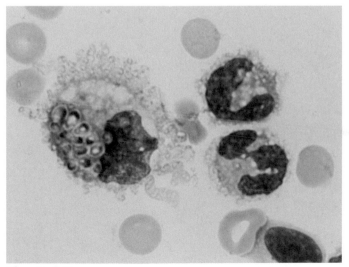

**Figure 8-3**
Buffy coat film from a dog. A large macrophage contains phagocytozed *Histoplasma* organisms.

# 9

# Lymphocytes

# OVERVIEW
## Origin

Peripheral blood lymphocytes originate either in the bone marrow or thymus.

In healthy dogs and cats, circulating lymphocytes (Figures 9-1A, B, and C) are approximately 70% thymus derived (T-lymphocytes) and approximately 30% bone marrow derived (B lymphocytes).

Unlike granulocytes and monocytes which move unidirectionally from bone marrow to blood to tissue, blood lymphocytes recirculate. The pattern is blood to lymph node to lymph and back to blood.
> ► Transit time in the blood during each circuit is estimated to be 8 to 12 hours.

Recirculating lymphocytes are long-lived cells which survive for months to years.

## Function

Lymphocytes are the cells of the specific immune system.
> ► B lymphocytes differentiate into plasma cells (Figure 9-2) which produce antibodies (humoral immunity).
> ► T lymphocytes are responsible for cellular immunity through the formation and release of molecules known collectively as cytokines.

Peripheral blood lymphocytes serve as the memory cells of the immune system.
> ► As they recirculate, lymphocytes monitor for the presence of antigens to which they have been previously sensitized.
> ► When lymphocytes activated by such contact enter lymph nodes, they can initiate both the cellular and humoral immune response through selective clonal expansion.

# QUANTITY
## Lymphopenia

Lymphopenia is a reduction in the number of circulating lymphocytes.

Causes of lymphopenia include:
> ► High circulating levels of glucocorticoids (stress, Cushing's disease).
> – Degree of lymphopenia is mild – counts between 750/$\mu$l and 1000/$\mu$l.
> – Counts lower than 750/$\mu$l suggest other causes.

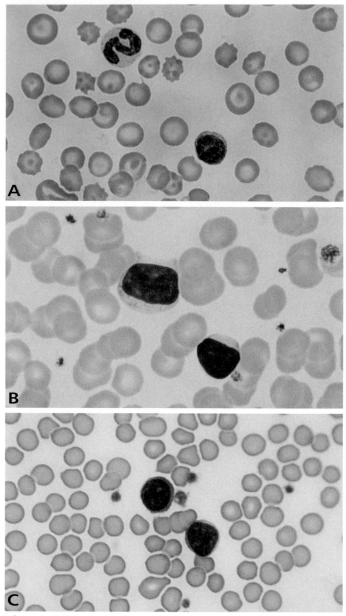

**Figure 9-1**

Normal lymphocytes. Lymphocytes in the dog and cat are the same size or smaller than a neutrophil. **A** and **B**, Canine lymphocytes have a scant amount of light blue cytoplasm with an eccentric, round, nucleus that has a dark, smooth chromatin. **C.** Feline lymphocytes are similar to those in the dog (A and C 100x, B 120x).

▶ Disruption of lymphatic recirculation (chylous effusions).
  – Counts can be very low (200/μl or less).
  – Often accompanied by decreased plasma protein.
▶ Lymphosarcoma
  – Lymphopenia can result from the inability of recirculating lymphocytes to migrate through effaced nodes.
  – Lymphopenia is as common in cases of lymphosarcoma as is lymphocytosis.

## Lymphocytosis

Lymphocytosis is an increase in the number of circulating lymphocytes.

Causes include:
▶ Excitement (physiologic lymphocytosis in cats only)
  – Physiologic lymphocytosis results from increased circulating epinephrine which causes increased blood flow and washes marginated lymphocytes back into circulation.
  – Lymphocyte counts can reach up to 20,000/μl.
  – Lymphocyte morphology and red cell measures are normal.
▶ Antigenic stimulation
  – Inflammatory conditions are often associated with antigenic stimulation. Over time, lymphocytosis and elevated globulins may result.
  – Many lymphocytes are reactive (see morphology below).
  – Vaccinations may cause lymphocytosis, often with many reactive forms.
▶ Lymphosarcoma/lymphocytic leukemia
  – Lymphocytosis is generally a late event.
  – Usually accompanied by marked nonregenerative anemia.
  – Thrombocytopenia and neutropenia may also be present.
  – Large numbers of circulating lymphocytes may be neoplastic lymphoblasts – large (20 μ or more) cells with lacy nuclear chromatin and   prominent large nucleoli.

# MORPHOLOGY
## Normal

Normal lymphocyte morphology is similar in dogs and cats.

Features of normal lymphocytes include (See Figure 9-1):
- ► Size – 9-12 $\mu$
- ► Nucleus – round, eccentric, clumped chromatin
- ► Cytoplasm – scant rim, pale blue

## Activated (Antigen-Stimulated) Lymphocytes

Antigen-stimulated lymphocytes are also known as reactive lymphocytes, immunocytes, or blast transformed lymphocytes.

Reactive lymphocytes represent an appropriate response to antigenic stimulation (Figure 9-3).

Morphologically similar in dogs and cats.

Antigen-stimulated B cells cannot be differentiated from antigen-stimulated T cells on the basis of morphology. However, differentiated B-lymphocytes are morpholicaly distinct and are recognized as plasma cells (Figure 9-2).

Morphology of reactive lymphocytes is highly variable from cell to cell. In general, features include:
- ► Size – 15-20 $\mu$
- ► Nucleus – large, reticular chromatin pattern. Nucleoli may be present.
- ► Cytoplasm – abundant, light to deep blue. Pale perinuclear zones may be present.

## Atypical Lymphocytes

Atypical lymphocytes are an abnormal finding (Table 9-1)

Atypical lymphocytes may be present in both infectious and neoplastic diseases and are therefore a nonspecific finding (Figures 9-4, 9-5, and 9-6).

Morphologic features include:
- ► Usually large
- ► Indented or clefted nuclei (termed Reiderform)
- ► Unusually large cytoplasmic azurophilic granules.

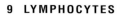

**Figure 9-2**
Plasma cells. B lymphocytes differentiate into plasma cells. These cells have an eccentric round nucleus, clumped chromatin, and blue cytoplasm that contains a focal clear zone (100x).

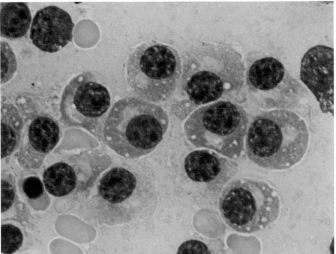

**Figure 9-3**
Reactive lymphocytes. Antigenic stimulation produces morphologic changes in canine **(A)** and feline **(B)** lymphocytes. Reactive lymphocytes are larger than a neutrophil, vary in size, and have dark blue cytoplasm. Nuclei are rounded with a reticular chromatin and remnants of nucleoli (100x).

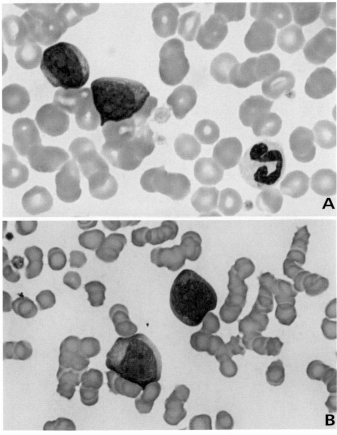

**TABLE 9-1  A Guide to Laboratory Features of Lymphocyte Abnormalities**

| Change | Classification | Mechanism | Occurence | Morphology | Other Findings | Comments |
|---|---|---|---|---|---|---|
| Decreased (Lymphopenia) | Corticosteroid or stress Induced | | Common | Normal | | Usually mild, seek other cause if <750/μl |
| | Disruption of recirculation | Sequestration in chylous effusions | Infrequent | Normal may occur | Hypoproteinemia | Lymphopenia is severe |
| | Lymphosarcoma | Trapping in neoplastic lymph nodes | Infrequent | Normal or occasional atypical lymphocyte | | Lymphopenia is as common with lymphosarcoma as lymphocytosis |
| Increased (Lymphocytosis) | Excitement – CATS ONLY | Marginated lymphocytes move into circulations | Common | Normal | Red Cell measures normal | Counts can reach up to 20,000/μl |
| | Antigenic stimulation | Clonal expansion response to antigenic stimulation | Common | Reactive (immunoblasts) | | May be seen 1-2 weeks after vaccination |
| | Lymphosarcoma | Neoplastic multiplication | Infrequent | Abnormal – large, lacy nuclei; prominent nucleoli | Marked non-regenerative anemia common | Lymphocytosis usually develops late in disease |

**Figure 9-4**
Canine atypical lymphocyte. The lymphocyte is larger than a neutrophil with a cleaved irregular nucleus that has reticulated chromatin (100x).

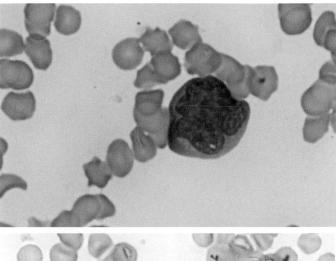

**Figure 9-5**
Feline atypical lymphocytes. The cells are round with abundant blue cytoplasm, large discrete irregular purple cytoplasmic granules, and oval nuclei with clumped chromatin. These cells are typical of large granular lymphoma in the cat (100x).

**Figure 9-6**
Canine lymphocytic leukemia. Numerous large lymphocytes are noted that have an abundant light blue cytoplasm, reticulated chromatin, and prominent nucleoli (100x).

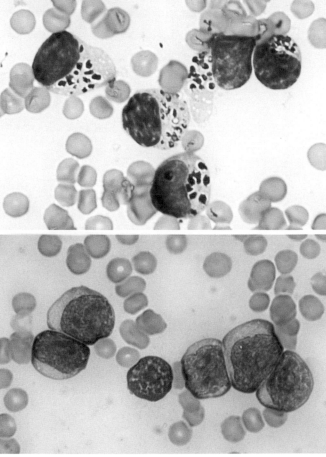

# 10
## Platelets

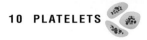

# OVERVIEW

Function and physiology

▶ Platelets are essential for normal hemostasis and perform four distinct functions:

- Maintenance of vascular integrity by sealing minor endothelial deficiencies.
- Helping to arrest bleeding by the formation of platelet plugs following endothelial constriction.
- Contributing membrane lipid procoagulant activity to facilitate secondary hemostasis (coagulation) and fibrin formation.
- Promoting vascular healing through platelet derived growth factor (PDGF).
  - Stimulates endothelial cell migration and smooth muscle production.

▶ Platelets are involved in the initial phase of wound repair through growth factors including PDGF.

- Rapid cell to cell interactions and release of soluble mediators stimulate mitogenesis of smooth muscle cells and fibroblasts.

▶ Platelets play an essential role in inflammation through cell to cell interaction and the release of soluble mediators.

- Platelets release vasoactive substances such as serotonin and also modulate neutrophil function.

Production

▶ Platelets are produced in the bone marrow from megakaryocytes.

- Formed by megakaryocytic cytoplasmic demarcation.
- Released directly into the venous blood vessels surrounding the marrow hematopoietic space.

▶ Thrombopoietin

- Regulates the development of megakaryocytes from hemopoietic stem cells.
- Appears to be involved only in the late development of megakaryocytes and the release of platelets from megakaryocytes.
- Concentration is inversely correlated with platelet numbers.
- The source of thrombopoietin is uncertain but appears to involve liver, endothelial cells, and fibroblasts.

▶ In the dog, two-thirds to three-quarters of all platelets are in the systemic circulation.

- The remainder exist as a splenic pool.

– This pool exchanges freely with the systemic circulation.

▶ The presence of a splenic pool in the cat is suspected but not defined.

Destruction

▶ Platelets have a variable but finite intravascular lifespan in the dog and cat of 3 to 7 days.

▶ Effete platelets are phagocytized by macrophages of the mononu clear phagocyte system.

– Anti-platelet antibody accelerates the destruction of platelets by macrophages leading to immune-mediated thrombocytopenia (see below).

# Laboratory Evaluation of Platelets

Examination of the complete hemogram is essential.

▶ Must establish whether thrombocytopenia is an isolated finding or associated with anemia or leukopenia

– If thrombocytopenia appears to be an isolated finding, repeat the count to confirm.

– The peripheral smear should be checked for platelet morpho-logic abnormalities, polychromatophilia, neutropenia, lym-phopenia, spherocytosis (not easily recognized in the cat), other red cell shape changes, or abnormal or unidentifiable cells.

Reticulated Platelet Count

▶ Reticulated platelets are immature with high ribonucleic acid content.

▶ Counting these platelets requires special stains and instrumentation.

▶ The number of reticulated platelets is useful in differentiating platelet destruction/consumption from decreased production.

Buccal Mucosal Bleeding Time (BMBT)

▶ A test to determine adequacy of endothelial function and platelet function.

▶ More sensitive test of platelet function than endothelial function

▶ Do not perform on patients with platelet counts < 75,000 per microliter.

Mean Platelet Volume (MPV)

▶ Estimated platelet size; similar to red cell size and mean cell volume (MCV)

– Inversely proportional to platelet number

▶ MPV in the dog is 6.1–10 femtoliters

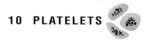
▶ MPV in the cat is 12–18 femtoliters

▶ Increase in MPV is suggestive of responsive thrombopoiesis

  – Occurs with secondary platelet destruction, some myeloproliferative diseases, and hyperthyroidism.

  – Artifactual increases in MPV arise when platelets are exposed to EDTA, cooled to room temperature or refrigerated, or if there is delayed exposure to anticoagulant.

  – Changes in MPV are minimized when blood is collected in citrate anticoagulant and kept at 37 degrees C until analyzed.

▶ Decreases in MPV have been reported in:

  – Dogs with early immune-mediated thrombocytopenia.

  – Bone marrow failure

Platelet Distribution Width (PDW)

▶ A value provided by some automated particle counters.

▶ Index of variation in platelet size (similar to red cell distribution width – RDW)

▶ PDW is a useful adjunct to smear evaluation of platelets.

▶ Examination of the PDW histogram may reveal the presence of abnormally sized platelets, either small or large (see morphology).

# MORPHOLOGY
## Normal Morphology: Dog
Shape:

  ▶ Discoid, oval, slightly elongated, slightly biconvex or flat with an even contour (Figure 10-1).

Romanowsky (Wright's or modified Wright's) stain:

  ▶ Central cluster of fine azurophilic granules surrounded by a pale blue matrix enclosed in a delicate membrane.

  ▶ Some platelets appear agranular or have only a few granules.

Size:

  ▶ 2.2-3.7 microns in diameter and 0.5 microns thick (approximately 1/10th the size of an erythrocyte).

  ▶ Young platelets are often large macroplatelets (megathrombocytes) (Figure 10-2).

Single platelets are most common. Small groups may be observed.

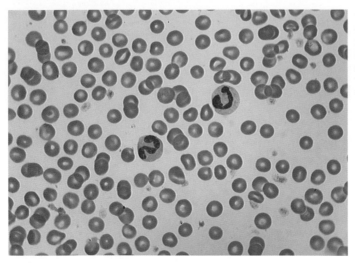

**Figure 10-1**
Canine platelets. Small round to oval, light blue, anucleated cells with a central cluster of purple granules. (50x).

## Normal Morphology: Cat

Feline platelets are morphologically similar to those of other domestic animals.

Shape:
- ► Small spherical bodies (Figure 10-3)
  - Sometimes appear as elongated structures
- ► Tend to clump, often resulting in amorphous masses (Figure 10-4)

Romanowsky stain:
- ► Central cluster of purple azurophilic granules surrounded by a pale blue background and enclosed in a delicate membrane.

Size:
- ► Variable
- ► Giant forms equal to the size of red blood cells are often observed in normal animals.

## Abnormal Morphology: Dog

Activated canine platelets have a spider-like appearance with small cytoplasmic pseudopodia.
- ► May form small clumps or an agglutinated mass (Figure 10-5). Large platelet masses are generally found on the feathered edge of push preparations (Figure 10-4).

Microplatelets
- ► When they predominate, they suggest an early immune-mediated event (immune-mediated thrombocytopenia) (Figures 10-6)

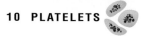

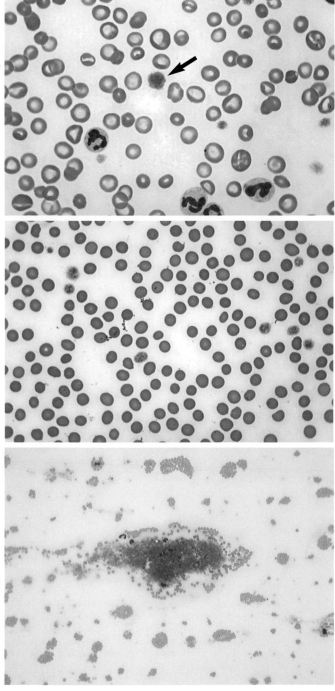

**Figure 10-2**
Canine platelets exhibiting platelet anisocytosis. Large purple platelet in center of field (arrow) is a young platelet. These are occasionally observed in normal canine blood smears (50x).

**Figure 10-3**
Normal feline platelets and red blood cells. Platelet size can be normally variable (anisocytosis) in feline blood smears (50x).

**Figure 10-4**
Large clump of feline platelets (center). Note size of the platelet clump as compared to the relatively tiny dark white cells at the periphery of the clump. Also note red cell clumps. These are typical of platelet and red cell appearance at the feathered edge of feline blood smears. Platelet clumping in cats could affect validity of both platelet and white cell counts (10x).

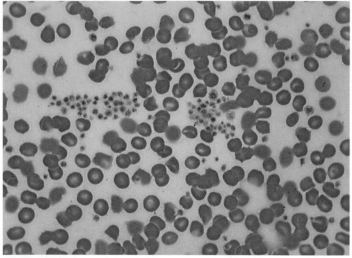

**Figure 10-5**
Clumped canine platelets (center) generally indicative of poor *ex vivo* anticoagulation (50x).

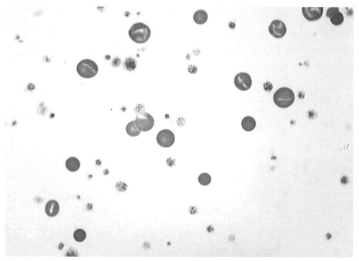

**Figure 10-6**
Canine blood smear from immune-mediated hemolytic anemia patient. Platelet numbers appear increased and platelet anisocytosis is evident. The tiny platelets are microplatelets suggesting the immune activity also involves the platelets. Large blue-red blood cells are immature red cells (polychromatophils). The small red cells without obvious central pallor are spherocytes (50x).

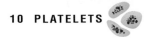

Platelet anisocytosis and numerous macroplatelets suggest marrow release of young platelets.

▶ Often observed in responsive thrombocytopenias (Figures 10-7, 10-8 and 10-9).

Notable numbers of elongated, cigar-shaped platelets suggest focal or generalized systemic hemorrhage.

▶ Further clinical investigation is warranted, such as determination of occult fecal or urinary blood or examination of body cavities, mucous membranes and hairless areas for evidence of hemorrhage.

Poorly granular platelets or platelets with few large granules suggest developmental abnormalities.

▶ Bone marrow examination is recommended.

Large granules must be examined as potential inclusions such as those associated with *Ehrlichia platys* (Figure 10-10).

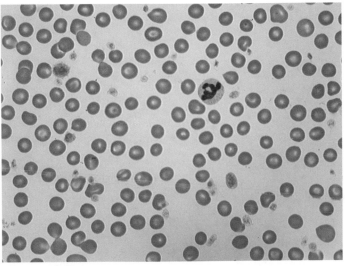

**Figure 10-7**
Canine blood smear. Platelet anisocytosis is evident. Large macroplatelet is in upper left quadrant. Large oval platelet is in lower right quadrant. These findings are associated with both increased platelet turnover and probable microhemorrhage (50x).

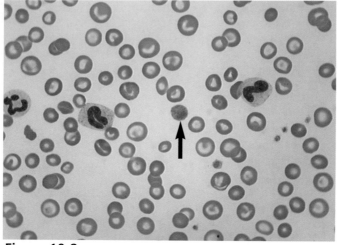

## Figure 10-8

Canine blood smear in responsive anemia. Do not confuse the immature blue red cells (polychromatophils) with the large blue granular platelet in the center of the field (arrow). Platelet numbers appear reduced and the large platelet (macroplatelet) could be indicative of increased platelet turnover in this situation (50x).

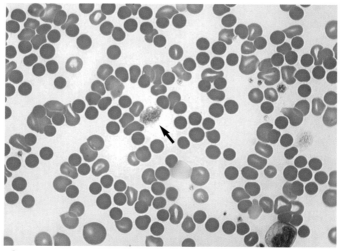

## Figure 10-9

Canine blood smear in immune-mediated hemolytic anemia and thrombocytopenia. Platelet numbers are reduced and a large blue granular cell (arrow) is a macroplatelet suggesting increased platelet turnover in this thrombocytopenic situation. Small dark red blood cells without central pallor throughout field are spherocytes (50x).

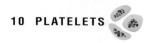

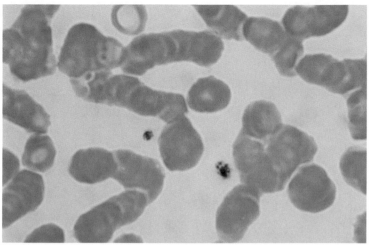

**Figure 10-10**
Canine blood smear. The platelet located at lower center contains
*Ehrlichia platys* morula (100x).

## Abnormal Morphology: Cat

Poorly granulated platelets or platelets with large granules suggest
developmental defects (Figure 10-11).

▶ Bone marrow examination is recommended.

Elongated forms or macroplatelets may be encountered in nonthrom-
bocytopenic cats.

## QUANTITY
## Normal

For both dogs and cats, 10-12 platelet per 1000x (oil immersion) field
are typical of a normal count.

In the normal dog, platelets circulate at a concentration of approximately
200,000/µl to 600,000/µl.

In the cat, platelet numbers are 300,000/µl to 800,000/µl.

▶ Excitement in cats results in sudden increases in platelet counts
with normal morphology.

▶ A decrease in platelet counts can be seen in splenectomized cats.
Morphology remains normal.

Feline platelets are prone to clumping.

▶ Produces inaccurately low platelet counts

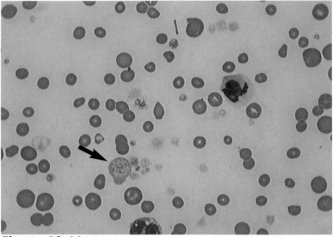

**Figure 10-11**
Feline blood smear in anemic patient. Note large blue-red cells
(polychromatophils) throughout the field. Platelet anisocytosis is
extreme with a bizarre macroplatelet in lower left quadrant
(arrow) suggesting developmental defect and need for bone
marrow examination (50x).

► Automated cell counters that rely on impedance may count
platelets as WBCs resulting in artifactually increased WBC
counts (see Chapter 3).

# Decreased Platelet Count (Thrombocytopenia)
## Clinical Signs of Thrombocytopenia
The clinical hallmark of thrombocytopenia is the occurrence of petechiae.
Petechiae

► Reflect capillary or postcapillary venule bleeding.

► Usually occur at sites of increased intravascular pressure.

– Lower abdomen

– Oral or genital mucosae

– Axillary or inguinal friction sites

Large coalescing petechiae are called purpura.

► Purpura are not usually palpable (skin texture, thickness are normal).

► Palpable purpura suggest an underlying systemic vasculitis.

Ecchymosis, or bruising, is also associated with primary hemostatic defects.

Clinical signs of bleeding can be seen in any thrombocytopenic patient.

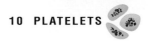

## TABLE 10-1  Causes of Thrombocytopenia

| Type | Disorder | Cause |
|---|---|---|
| Platelet production defect | Aplasia, hypoplasia, pancytopenia | Cytotoxic drugs; idiopathic |
| | Marrow infiltration, pancytopenia | Drugs, infection including viral infections |
| | Ineffective megakaryocytopoiesis | Myelodysplastic syndrome |
| Accelerated platelet removal | Immune destruction | Autoantibodies; antibodies to drugs, infection |
| | Nonimmunologic removal | DIC, vasculitis, severe bleeding, neoplasia, infection |
| Platelet Sequestration | Hypersplenism | Enlarged spleen from numerous causes |

▶ The rapidity with which thrombocytopenia occurs affects the platelet number at which clinical signs occur.

– Rapid platelet destruction leads to hemorrhagic tendencies at much higher platelet counts.

▶ If platelets are also dysfunctional, clinical signs occur with only modest reductions in numbers.

– Often occurs with rickettsial diseases.

Patients with concomitant illnesses and thrombocytopenia bleed more.

### Causes of Thrombocytopenia

There are four major mechanisms which result in thrombocytopenia (Table 10-1).

▶ Abnormal platelet production

▶ Accelerated platelet removal

▶ Abnormal distribution of platelets

▶ Some combination of the above

### Abnormal Platelet Production (Rare)

Virtually always accompanied by another cytopenia such as anemia and/or neutropenia.

Platelet production defects include:

▶ Pure megakaryocytic hypoplasia

– Immune or infectious etiologies

► Marrow panhypoplasia
  – Drug, infectious, or toxic etiologies
► Dysthrombopoiesis (myelodysplasia or megakaryocytic leukemia)
  – Diagnosis requires bone marrow aspirate at least; marrow core biopsy is recommended.
  – Multiple aspirates on different days may be required.

Infectious causes include:
► Ehrlichiosis
► Feline leukemia virus (FeLV) infection
► Feline immunodeficiency virus (FIV) infection

Vaccination-induced interference with platelet production has been reported.
► In dogs: measles, distemper, parvoviral vaccinations
► In cats: feline panleukopenia vaccination

Drug-induced suppression of thrombopoiesis
► Usually affects other cell lines also.
► Neutropenia usually occurs at day 5 and thrombocytopenia at days 8-10 after exposure to drug.
► Anemia is not usually seen because of longer red cell lifespan.
► Commonly implicated drugs are estrogen, sulfadiazine, and non-steroidal anti-inflammatory drugs.

## Accelerated Platelet Removal (Common)
Causes of accelerated platelet removal include immune mediated thrombocytopenia, alloimmune thrombocytopenia, and secondary non-immune thrombocytopenia (See Figures 10-8 and 10-9).
► Both primary and secondary immune mediated thrombocytopenias occur
► Primary immune-mediated thrombocytopenia
  – Is most common in dogs with some breed predisposition
    • Cocker Spaniels
    • English Sheepdogs
    • German Shepherds
    • Poodles
  – Is associated with the presence of antiplatelet antibodies which cause accelerated destruction by the mononuclear phagocyte system
  – May also be associated with anti-megakaryocyte antibodies which impair thrombopoiesis.

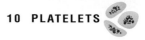

– Is associated with variable clinical signs including hemorrhage from the mucous membranes, skin, genitalia, nose, or gastrointestinal tract.
  ◆ Many severely thrombocytopenic patients remain asymptomatic.
– Laboratory findings in primary immune-mediated thrombocytopenia include:
  ◆ Severe thrombocytopenia, often less than 30,000/μl.
  ◆ The presence of increased proportions of small or large platelets.
  ◆ Megakaryocytic hyperplasia in the marrow if antibodies are directed against circulating platelets, reduced numbers of megakaryocytes if the disease is marrow directed.
– Establishing the diagnosis is mainly by exclusion.
  ◆ Rule out pseudothrombocytopenia due to platelet clumping or EDTA anticoagulation.
  ◆ Splenomegaly suggests a secondary process.
  ◆ Anemia suggests a concurrent disease process.
  ◆ Drug exposure, infection, recent vaccination neoplasia, or previous transfusion must be considered.
– Special tests include:
  ◆ Serology and polymerase chain reaction (PCR) tests for rickettsial agents.
  ◆ Tests for systemic immune-mediated disease such as antinuclear antibodies, rheumatoid factor, lupus erythematosus cells, and red or white cell-associated antibody tests.
  ◆ Antiplatelet antibody assays are useful but require fresh platelets and specialized instrumentation.
  ◆ The direct megakaryocyte immunofluorescence assay is a good test but requires special technical expertise and air-dried bone marrows.
▶ Secondary immune-mediated thrombocytopenia
  – Is the most common cause of canine thrombocytopenia and the most common canine hemostatic disorder.
  – Is associated with underlying conditions including
    ◆ Systemic autoimmune disease
      ✓ systemic lupus erythematosus (SLE)
      ✓ immune-mediated hemolytic anemia
      ✓ rheumatoid arthritis
      ✓ pemphigus
      ✓ juvenile-onset polyarthritis of Akitas

- Neoplasia
  - ✓ multicentric or metastatic
  - ✓ hematologic
- Infectious diseases
  - ✓ FeLV, FIV in cats
  - ✓ Ehrlichiosis
  - ✓ Rocky Mountain spotted fever
- Vaccination with modified live virus distemper vaccines (transient)
- Protozoal infections such as leishmaniasis and babesiosis
- Dirofilariasis
- Histoplasmosis
- Immune-complex vasculitis

Alloimmune thrombocytopenia
- ▶ Occurs when maternal antibodies to paternal antigens are transferred across the placenta or in colostrum and cause platelet destruction in the neonate.
- ▶ Is not reported in dogs and cats.
- ▶ Post-transfusion purpura has been described in dogs receiving DEA1 incompatible erythrocytes, or plasma.
  - – The resultant thrombocytopenia appears to resolve within hours.

Secondary nonimmune thrombocytopenia
- ▶ Causes of secondary nonimmune thrombocytopenia include disseminated intravascular coagulation, thrombotic thrombocytopenic purpura, and hemolytic uremic syndrome.
- ▶ Disseminated intravascular coagulation (DIC)
  - – Occurs secondary to systemic inflammation (acute, subacute, chronic).
  - – Is associated with vascular damage, sepsis, release of tissue thromboplastin from diseased or neoplastic tissue.
- ▶ Thrombotic thrombocytopenic purpura
  - – Severe thrombocytopenia, intravascular hemolysis with schistocytosis, and neurologic signs.
- ▶ Hemolytic uremic syndrome
  - – Severe thrombocytopenia, intravascular hemolysis with schistocytosis, and renal dysfunction.

## Abnormal Platelet Distribution

Abnormal platelet distribution is associated with hypersplenism and endotoxemia.

Hypersplenism
▶ A pathologic condition in which a large proportion of circulating platelets become sequestered in the spleen.
▶ One or more cytopenias is usually present.
▶ Splenomegaly is sometimes present.

Endotoxemia may cause splenic pooling of platelets

## Drug-Induced Thrombocytopenia

Decreased platelet production, accelerated platelet removal, and platelet sequestration can all be associated with the use of various pharmaceuticals.

Implicated drugs include
▶ Antibiotics
▶ Antimicrobial agents
▶ Anticonvulsants
▶ Anti-inflammatory agents
▶ Chemotherapeutic agents
▶ Antiviral drugs
▶ Diuretics

Drug-induced thrombocytopenias may be marrow-mediated or peripherally mediated.

Drug-induced marrow-mediated thrombocytopenia
▶ Bone marrow suppression
– Most often associated with direct cytotoxic effects on progenitor cells.
▶ Immune-mediated drug-induced destruction of megakaryocytes has been reported in the dog.

Drug-induced peripherally-mediated thrombocytopenia
▶ Can be either immune-mediated or nonimmune.
▶ Immune-mediated drug-related thrombocytopenia
– Some drugs provoke an immune response against unadulterated platelets such as methyldopa, levodopa, and gold.

- Other drugs provoke antibody formation against drug-platelet antigen complexes such as heparin and quinine.
- Still other drugs cause immune-mediated thrombocytopenia after prolonged drug therapy or the reintroduction of a previously used drug.
  - Secondary exposure results in antibody formation
  - Drug absorbed or adsorbed to the platelet surface
  - Platelet destroyed as an innocent bystander by immune activity

# Increased Platelet Count (Thrombocytosis)
## Mechanisms of Thrombocytosis
There are three categories of thrombocytosis.
- Essential thrombocytosis (primary bone marrow disorder)
- Secondary to disease
- Physiological

## Essential Thrombocythemia
- Is a rare myeloproliferative disorder.
- Is characterized by persistent primary thrombocytosis.
- Synonyms
  - Idiopathic thrombocythemia
  - Primary hemorrhagic thrombocythemia
  - Thrombasthenia
- Has been associated with bleeding or thombosis.
- Described in middle-aged to older dogs and in one cat.
  - Platelets are often dysfunctional (thrombocytopathic) in aggregation and adhesion studies.
  - MPV is usually within reference range.
- Dogs are presented with both nonregenerative and regenerative anemia, occasional hypogranular macroplatelets, basophilia, and spurious hyperkalemia.

## Secondary (reactive) Thrombocytosis
- Characterized by transiently increased platelet counts in patients with conditions other than myeloproliferative disorders (Figures 10-12).
  - Neoplasia
    - Lymphoma, hematologic neoplasia, melanoma, mast cell

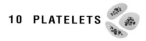

neoplasia, adenocarcinoma, mesothelioma, central nervous
system neoplasia.
- Gastrointestinal disorders
  ◆ Pancreatitis, hepatitis, inflammatory bowel disease, colitis
- Immune-mediated disease
- Blood loss/hemorrhage
  ◆ Iron deficiency, trauma, and surgical trauma
- Fractures
- Drug therapy
  ◆ Glucocorticoids and antineoplastic drugs
- Postsplenectomy in dogs

## Physiologic Thrombocytosis

▶ Results from increased mobilization of platelets from splenic and
nonsplenic (perhaps pulmonary) pools.

▶ Transient as the result of exercise or epinephrine injection.

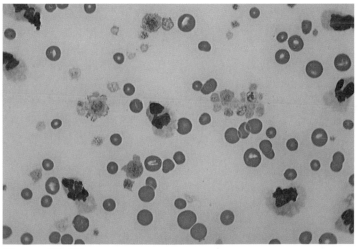

**Figure 10-12**
Feline blood smear exhibiting thrombocytosis and responsive anemia. Platelet clump is at right center. Three bizarre macro platelets
are found in the left half of the field from top to bottom indicating
platelet developmental abnormalities and the need for bone marrow
examination (50x).

# PLATELET FUNCTION DISORDERS (THROMBOCYTOPATHIA OR THROMBOPATHIA)

Suggested by clinical hemorrhage and prolonged buccal mucosal bleeding time despite a platelet count >100,000 per microliter (Table 10-2).

Clinical signs:
- ▶ Bleeding from mucosal surfaces
- ▶ Melena
- ▶ Hematuria
- ▶ Epistaxis
- ▶ Cutaneous ecchymoses
- ▶ Prolonged or excessive bleeding at venipuncture, trauma, or surgery sites
- ▶ Hallmarks of systemic bleeding disorder due to platelet malfunction:
  - Bleeding at more than one location
  - Multiple ecchymoses
  - Previous bleeding history
  - Bleeding is persistent or recurring.
  - The amount of bleeding is much greater than anticipated.
  - There is no "apparent" history of trauma.
  - Platelet count is within reference range.
  - Activated partial thromboplastin time (APTT), prothrombin time (PT), and fibrinogen concentration are appropriate.
  - Tests to define or diagnose DIC are negative.

Buccal Mucosal Bleeding Time (BMBT)
- ▶ Utilizes a "bleeding time device," a guillotine-like device that creates an incision standardized in terms of length and depth.
- ▶ Preferred to any other "bleeding time test".
- ▶ Ideally performed on a nontranquilized or nonanesthetized patient.
  - A somewhat loose gauze tie (in preference to fingers) holds the folded back upper lip in place to expose the buccal mucosa.
- ▶ As blood seeps from the incision, paper toweling is used to soak up the blood.
  - Use care not to touch the incision site.
  - The time from incision to cessation of bleeding is the BMBT.
  - The reference interval for the dog and cat: 1.8 to 4.2 minutes
  - Most patients will have times closer to the lower end of the interval.

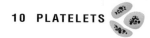

## TABLE 10-2 Classification of Platelet Function Defects (Thrombocytopathy)

| Type | Characteristic | Cause |
|------|----------------|-------|
| Acquired | Production of abnormal, platelets | Myeloproliferative disease, myelodysplasia |
| | Dysfunction of normal platelets | Systemic disease (uremia liver disease, DIC, myeloma), non-steroidal antiinflammatory drugs, dextran, colloids |
| Congenital | Deficiency of plasma factor | Deficiency or abnormality of von Willebrand factor |
| | Membrane abnormalities | Thrombasthenia |
| | Platelet granule abnormalities | Deficiency or absence of platelet dense granules |

# Causes of Platelet Dysfunction (Thrombocytopathy)

Platelet dysfunction can be acquired or inherited.

## *Acquired Platelet Dysfunction*

► May manifest as reduced platelet function (hyporesponsiveness) or enhanced platelet function (hyperresponsiveness).

## *Acquired Hyporesponsiveness with Bleeding Tendencies*

► Causes include:
  – Uremia
  – Dysproteinemia
  – Infectious agents
    ◆ Ehrlichia canis
    ◆ Feline leukemia virus
  – Snake venom
  – Hepatic disease
  – Neoplasia
    ◆ Especially leukemia or myeloproliferative disease
  – Drugs (Table 10-3)
    ◆ Anti-inflammatory agents including aspirin, ibuprofen, acetaminophen, flunixin, butazolidine
    ◆ Antibiotics including penicillin and cephalothin
    ◆ Calcium channel blockers – diltiazem, nifedipine, verapamil
    ◆ Dextrans
    ◆ Colloids

## Acquired Hyperresponsiveness or Prothrombotic States
► Causes include:
  – Diabetes mellitus
  – Hyperadrenocorticism – Cushing's disease
  – Nephrotic syndrome
  – Hormone treatment – treatment with erythropoietin or patients with severe responsive anemias may have hyperreactive platelets
  – Neoplasia – both sarcomas and carcinomas have been implicated in enhanced platelet activity
  – Infectious agents
    ◆ Feline infectious peritonitis
    ◆ Heartworm disease

## Inherited Platelet Dysfunction
Inherited platelet functional disorders have been described in many breeds of dogs and in cats.

### Von Willebrand Disease (vWd)
► The most common canine hereditary bleeding disorder.
► Three subtype classifications which are dependent on the severity of clinical signs, mode of inheritance, and biochemical abnormalities of von Willebrand factor protein (vWf).
  – Type 1 vWd has been observed in many canine breeds and in cats. There is a mild bleeding tendency.
  – Type 2 vWd is observed in German shorthaired and wirehaired pointers. There is a moderate bleeding tendency.
  – Type 3 vWd is observed in the Scottish terrier, Chesapeake Bay retriever, and Shetland sheep dog. There is a moderate bleeding tendency. Von Willebrand factor is usually 0 percent.
► The pathognomonic feature of vWd is lack of functional of von Willebrand factor (vWf).
  – Causes abnormal primary hemostasis
► Clinical signs
  – Mucosal hemorrhage, cutaneous bruising, and prolonged bleeding from sites of trauma or surgery.
  – Bleeding can be mild (common) to severe (relatively uncommon).
  – Bleeding is exacerbated by concurrent thrombocytopenia, disease conditions that impair platelet function, and the use of nonsteroidal anti-inflammatory drugs.

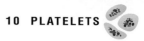

## TABLE 10-3 Drugs Affecting Platelet Function

Anesthetics
    General – Halothane
    Local – Procaine
Antibiotics
    Cephalosporins – Cefazolin
    Penicillins – Ampicillin
Anticoagulants – Heparin
Antihistamines – Chlorpheniramine
Cardiovascular drugs – Propanolol, Verapamil
Foods and food additives – Ethanol, onions
Nonsteroidal anti-inflammatory drugs – Aspirin, Phenylbutazone
Oncologic drugs – Daunorubicin
Plasma expanders – Heta starch, Dextrans
Miscellaneous drugs – Chlorpromazine

▶ Many breeds of purebred dogs are affected. Affected mixed breed dogs have been observed.

▶ Diagnosis: The platelet count, APTT, PT, are normal but the BMBT is prolonged.
  – Definitive diagnosis requires specific assay of plasma vWf
    ◆ Canine and feline vWf are antigenically and functionally distinct from human vWf.
    ◆ Each laboratory should provide reference intervals for each species assayed. Quantitative values less than 50 percent are considered vWf deficient.
    ◆ Structural assays are utilized to subtype vWd.

### Canine Thrombasthenic Thrombopathia

▶ Is an autosomal inherited disorder in great Pyrenees and Otterhounds

▶ Clinical hemorrhage is associated with mucosal surfaces and is exacerbated by trauma and stress.

▶ Bleeding episodes may be associated with vaccination, hypothyroidism, or estrus.

### Basset Hound Thrombopathia

▶ Autosomal inheritance

▶ Often confused with vWd

▶ BMBT is prolonged

► Bleeding is usually associated with mucosal or cutaneous surfaces
► Similar defects have been observed in the American foxhound and in cats.

## Spitz Thrombopathia
► A variant of canine thrombasthenic thrombopathia
► Chronic epistaxis, gingival bleeding, and gastrointestinal bleeding

## Cocker Spaniel Bleeding Disorders
► Delta storage pool disease associated with moderate bleeding and abnormal platelet aggregation
► Cocker spaniels have numerous other hereditary hemostatic disorders including factor II (prothombin) deficiency and factor X deficiency
► Both are manifest by bleeding and prolonged APTT and PT

# 11

# Interpretation of the Hemogram

# INTRODUCTION

Hemograms consist of both quantitative data (total cell counts, differential cell counts, red cell indices, etc.) and qualitative data (blood film morphology). Proper interpretation depends on the integration of both.

Proper interpretation also depends upon the development of a systematic approach. For both quantitative and qualitative data, we recommend evaluation of white cells first, followed by red cells, and then platelets.

For all cell compartments, interpretation can be guided by asking and answering a series of well-designed questions.

## WHITE CELLS (Table 11-1)

Overview
- ▶ Quantitative data includes total white cell count and differential count
- ▶ Qualitative data is white cell morphology
- ▶ Key questions include:
  - Is there evidence of inflammation?
  - Is there evidence of stress?
  - Is there evidence of tissue necrosis?
  - Is there evidence of systemic hypersensitivity?
  - If inflammatory, can the response be classified as acute, chronic, or overwhelming?
  - Is there evidence of systemic toxemia?

Is there evidence of inflammation?
- ▶ Persistent eosinophilia, monocytosis, and a neutrophilic left shift (increased numbers of immature neutrophils), alone or in combination, suggest inflammation.
- ▶ Total white cell count merely reflects balance between marrow production and tissue utilization; in inflammation, total white cell counts may be low, normal, or high.
- ▶ Absolute neutrophilias of greater than 25,000/μl are also suggestive of inflammation.

Is there evidence of stress (high circulating levels of glucocorticords)?
- ▶ Stress typically results in mild lymphopenia (lymphocyte counts between 750/μl and 1500/μl).
- ▶ Eosinopenia, mild neutrophilia, and mild monocytosis may also be present but are less consistent and nonspecific.

## TABLE 11-1  General Patterns of Leukocyte Responses

| | WBC | Seg | Band | Lymph | Mono | Eos |
|---|---|---|---|---|---|---|
| Acute Inflammation | Increased | Increased | Increased | Decreased or no change | Variable | Variable |
| Chronic Inflammation | Increased or no change | Increased or no change | Increased or no change | Increased or no change | Increased | Variable |
| Overwhelming Inflammation | Decreased or no change | Decreased or no change | Increased | Decreased or no change | Variable | Variable |
| Excitement leukocytosis | Increased | Increased in dogs; increased or no change in cats | No change | No change in dogs; increased in cats | No change | No change |
| Stress leukogram | Increased | Increased | No change | Decreased | Increased or no change | Decreased or no change |

Is there evidence of tissue necrosis?
- ► Monocytosis indicates tissue necrosis and demand for phagocytosis. Monocytosis can occur with acute or chronic inflammation or necrosis.

Is there evidence of systemic hypersensitivity?
- ► Persistent eosinophilia and/or basophilia is an indicator of systemic hypersensitivity.
- ► Causes include:
  - – Parasitic diseases with a systemic component, eg., heartworms, flea bite dermatitis
  - – Allergic tracheobronchitis in dogs (pulmonary infiltrates with eosinophils)
  - – Feline asthma
  - – Allergic gastroenteritis
  - – Systemic mastocytosis
  - – Disseminated eosinophilic granuloma complex in cats
  - – Parasitic disease confined to the intestinal tract (eg., whip worms) does not cause eosinophilia!!

Can the inflammatory response be classified as acute, chronic, or overwhelming?
- ► In many cases, inflammatory leukograms cannot be further classified.
- ► In other cases, the differential cell count is typical of acute, chronic, or overwhelming inflammation.
- ► These typical patterns reflect changes in leukocyte kinetics, or the balance between white cell production in the marrow and white cell utilization in the tissues. These changes are controlled by chemotactic factors and cytokines.
- ► The typical acute inflammatory leukogram is characterized by neutrophilia with increased band cells (a regenerative left shift), lymphopenia, and variable monocytosis.
  - – Neutrophilia reflects a large bone marrow storage pool in dogs and cats and the movement of larger numbers of neutrophils from marrow into blood than are moving from blood into tissues
  - – The left shift suggests depletion of the marrow storage pool of neutrophils with the subsequent recruitment of younger cells into circulation.
  - – The lymphopenia reflects stress, a common accompaniment of acute inflammatory processes.
  - – When present, the monocytosis reflects demand for phagocytosis /tissue necrosis.

▶ There are two patterns typical of chronic inflammation:
 – Marked leukocytosis (50,000-120,000/μl) with marked neutrophilia and left shift, neutrophil toxicity, and monocytosis.
   ◆ Most commonly seen with severe focal suppurative lesions
   ◆ Usually accompanied by the anemia of inflammatory disease and hyperglobulinemia
 – Normal to slightly elevated white cell count characterized by normal to slightly elevated neutrophil counts, no left shift, normal lymphocyte counts, and monocytosis.
   ◆ The normal to slightly elevated neutrophil count reflects a new balance between marrow production and tissue demand. This balance results from expanded production of neutrophils by the bone marrow in response to cytokines (growth factors) released at the tissue site of injury.
   ◆ The lack of left shift reflects the fact that marrow production of neutrophils has expanded to meet increased tissue demand.
   ◆ The normal lymphocyte count reflects the counterbalancing effects of stress and antigenic stimulation on lymphocyte numbers.
   ◆ Monocytosis reflects demand for phagocytosis/tissue necrosis.
▶ The typical overwhelming inflammatory response is characterized by reduced neutrophil numbers, a left shift, lymphopenia, and variable monocytosis.
 – Reduced numbers of neutrophils suggest inability of marrow production to keep pace with tissue demand.
 – Left shift indicates depletion of marrow neutrophil storage pools.
 – Lymphopenia reflects stress.
 – When present, monocytosis indicates tissue necrosis/demand for phagocytosis.
Is there evidence of systemic toxemia?
▶ The presence of toxic neutrophils on the blood film indicates systemic toxemia (see neutrophil morphology).
 – Systemic toxemia is most commonly associated with bacterial infections.
 – However, other causes, such as extensive tissue necrosis, must also be considered.

# RED CELLS
Overview
 ▶ Quantitative data includes red cell count, hemoglobin, hemat-

ocrit, red cell indices (MCV, MCHC), and total protein.

– Red cell count, hemoglobin, and hematocrit are all measures of red cell mass.

– Total protein provides information about state of hydration. Elevations most commonly result from dehydration which can also falsely elevate indicators of red cell mass.

▶ Qualitative data is red cell morphology determined from the blood film.

▶ Key questions include:

– Is red cell mass increased (polycythemia), decreased (anemia), or normal?

– If decreased, is anemia regenerative or nonregenerative?

– If regenerative, is the mechanism blood loss or hemolysis?

– If nonregenerative, can the mechanism be determined without bone marrow evaluation?

– If red cell mass is increased, is the polycythemia relative or absolute?

– If polycythemia is absolute, is it primary or secondary?

Is red cell mass increased, decreased, or normal?

▶ Answered by evaluating the indicators of red cell mass.

If decreased, is the anemia regenerative or nonregenerative (Figure 11-1)?

▶ Evaluating the blood film is the critical first step in recognizing regenerative anemias. Increased numbers of polychromatophilic erythrocytes on the blood film suggests red cell regeneration.

▶ Regeneration is confirmed by doing absolute reticulocyte counts. In dogs and cats, absolute reticulocyte counts of greater than 80,000/$\mu$l indicate regeneration.

If regenerative, is the mechanism blood loss or hemolysis?

▶ History, signs, and physical exam are key to differentiation. Most causes of blood loss will be recognized in this way.

▶ Hemoglobinemia or hemoglobinuria indicate hemolysis.

▶ Very high reticulocyte counts (>200,000/$\mu$l) are highly suggestive of hemolysis.

▶ Where hemolysis is suspected, red cell morphology should be scrutinized for abnormal red cells which are characteristic of certain hemolytic disorders. These are described and illustrated elsewhere (see Chapter 4) but include:

– Spherocytes

– Heinz bodies

– Schistocytes

– Etiologic agents (*Haemobartonella, Babesia*)

– Ghost cells

– Eccentrocytes

If nonregenerative, can the mechanism be determined without bone marrow evaluation?

▶ The anemia of inflammatory disease is the most common anemia of dogs and cats and can be presumptively diagnosed from the hemogram. Characteristics include:

– Mild to moderate normocytic normochromic anemia

– An inflammatory leukogram

▶ Iron deficiency causes a characteristic microcytic hypochromic nonregenerative anemia which can be presumptively diagnosed from hemogram data and blood films.

▶ Megaloblastic anemias (nuclear maturation defect anemias) often have occasional giant red cells (macrocytes) in circulation. Megaloblasts (see Chapter 4) may also be present on blood films. Marrow confirmation is required.

▶ Myelofibrosis of the bone marrow causes nonregenerative anemia with the following characteristics:

– Poikilocytosis with dacryocytes and ovalocytes

– Leukopenia

– Variable platelet response. Marrow histopathologic confirmation is required.

▶ Nonregenerative anemias characterized by large numbers (>10/100 WBC counted) of nucleated red cells on blood films in the absence of polychromasia (an inappropriate nucleated red cell response) indicates bone marrow stromal damage. Causes are most likely:

– Lead poisoning in dogs

– FeLV infection in cats

▶ All other nonregenerative anemias have nonspecific hemogram findings and can only be further assessed via bone marrow evaluation.

If red cell mass is increased, is polycythemia relative or absolute?

▶ Relative polycythemia (due to dehydration) is the most common form. It is characterized by:

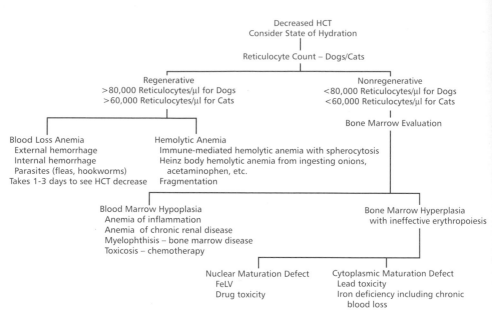

**Figure 11-1**
Interpretive approach to the evaluation of anemia.

- Increased red cell mass
- Increased total protein
- Serum chemical indicators of dehydration

▶ When relative polycythemia is ruled out, the remaining cases are absolute polycythemias.

If absolute, is polycythemia secondary or primary?
▶ Secondary polycythemia is associated with (caused by) a number of other diseases including:
- Cardiovascular disease
- Pulmonary disease
- Renal disease
- Renal neoplasms (primary or metastatic)
- Cushing's disease

▶ In the absence of such an underlying cause, polycythemia is considered to be primary (due to the myeloproliferative disorder polycythemia vera). Polycythemia vera is characterized by:
- Normal tissue oxygenation (normal arterial blood gas)
- Normal erythropoietin levels

# PLATELETS

Overview

▶ The quantitative platelet test is platelet number.

▶ The qualitative platelet test is platelet morphology.

▶ Key questions include:
  – If there is increased platelet count (thrombocytosis), is it reactive or primary?
  – If there is a decreased platelet count (thrombocytopenia), can the mechanism be determined?
  – If the platelet count is normal but there is evidence of bleeding, could it be the result of dysfunctional platelets (thrombocytopathy)?
  – Is platelet morphology abnormal?

If there is thrombocytosis, is it reactive or primary?

▶ Reactive thrombocytosis is seen secondarily with:
  – Splenectomy
  – Excitement
  – Exercise
  – Fractures
  – High circulating glucocorticoid levels
  – Post-blood loss (24 hours or more)
  – Myelofibrosis
  – Iron deficiency anemia

▶ Primary thrombocytosis is seen as a distinctive form of platelet leukemia or in association with other myeloproliferative disorders.

If there is a thrombocytopenia, can the mechanism be determined?

▶ Consumptive thrombocytopenias are associated with inflammation, DIC, and infectious diseases such as Ehrlichiosis and other tick-borne diseases. Features include:
  – Inflammatory leukogram
  – Mild to moderate thrombocytopenia (platelet counts generally greater than 50,000)
  – Schistocytes (in dogs)
  – Normal numbers of marrow precursors

▶ Sequestration thrombocytopenias are associated with hepatosplenomegaly

▶ Hypoproliferative thrombocytopenias are associated with reduced numbers of marrow precursors.

► Destructive thrombocytopenias are immune-mediated. They may occur alone or in combination with immune mediated hemolytic disease. Common features include:
  – Marked thrombocytopenia ($<50,000/\mu l$)
  – Normal to increased numbers of marrow precursors

If platelet count is normal but there is evidence of bleeding, could it be the result of thrombocytopathy?
► First rule out other causes of bleeding
  – Trauma
  – Coagulation defects (activated partial thromboplastin time, APTT, and prothrombin time, PT, are normal)
  – DIC – fibrinogen and fibrin split products are also within normal
► Run buccal mucosal bleeding time (BMBT)
  – If prolonged, consider thrombocytopathy as a possible (likely) cause

Is platelet morphology abnormal?
► The presence of significant numbers of small platelets (microplatelets) suggests the early phase of a possible immune-mediated thrombocytopenia
► Platelet anisocytosis characterized by significant numbers of enlarged platelets (macroplatelets) suggests increased marrow production of platelets. Commonly seen in responsive thrombocytopenias and regenerative anemias.
► Poorly granulated platelets with a few large granules suggest developmental abnormalities. Evaluate bone marrow.
► Excessively large granules in platelets should be examined as potential inclusions such as those associated with *Ehrlichia platys*.

# 12

# Case Studies

# NOTES

# CASE 1 Feline 8 Month Old Intact Male DSH

**History** Cat presented for castration and declaw surgery.

**Physical Examination** Normal temperature, pulse, and respiration (TPR). Cat is extremely fractious and is salivating profusely.

## Laboratory Data

|  | Patient | Reference Range |  | Patient | Reference Range |
|---|---|---|---|---|---|
| PCV % | 35 | (30-40) | WBC/ul | 26,500 | (5,500-19,500) |
| Hgb g/dl | 11.6 | (8.5-15) | Neutrophils | 13,250 | (2,500-12,500) |
| RBC x10⁶/ul | 7.6 | (5.2-10) | Band cells | --- | (0-300) |
| MCV fl | 46 | (39-55) | Lymphocytes | 12,455 | (1,500-7,000) |
| MCH pg | 15 | (13-17) | Monocytes | 795 | (0-850) |
| MCHC g/dl | 33 | (30-36) | Eosinophils | --- | (0-750) |
| TPP g/dl | 7.1 | (6.0-7.5) |  |  |  |
| Platelets | ADQ |  |  |  |  |

## Discussion/Interpretation

CBC reveals a marked lymphocytosis with a slight mature neutrophilia. Causes of lymphocytosis include chronic infection or inflammation, lymphocytic leukemia, and physiologic lymphocytosis. Examination of the blood film reveals numerous small lymphocytes. Lymphoblasts or atypical lymphocytes were not observed. Tests for FeLV and FIV were negative.

This is an example of a physiologic lymphocytosis and neutrophilia in a young, healthy, scared cat. Epinephrine release causes demargination of neutrophils and lymphocytosis. Both changes are transient and values return to normal within 1-2 hours.

# NOTES

## CASE 2  Canine 6 Year Old Castrated Male Dachshund

**History**  Back pain with posterior paresis for 2 days.

**Physical Examination**  Intervertebral disc protrusion at T13 – L1.

**Laboratory Data**

| | Patient | Reference Range | | Patient | Reference Range |
|---|---|---|---|---|---|
| PCV % | 40 | (37-55) | WBC/ul | 28,000 | (6,000-17,000) |
| Hgb g/dl | 13.3 | (12-18) | Neutrophils | 25,200 | (3,000-11,400) |
| RBC x10⁶/ul | 6.0 | (5.5-8.5) | Band cells | --- | (0-300) |
| MCV fl | 66 | (60-77) | Lymphocytes | 840 | (1,000-4,800) |
| MCH pg | 22 | (19-24) | Monocytes | 1,960 | (150-1,350) |
| MCHC g/dl | 33 | (32-36) | Eosinophils | --- | (100-750) |
| TPP g/dl | 7.5 | (6.0-7.5) | | | |
| Platelets | ADQ | | | | |

### Discussion/Interpretation

The leukogram reveals a lymphopenia, eosinopenia, and a leukocytosis due to a neutrophilia without a left shift and a monocytosis. These changes represent the effects of glucocorticoid therapy. The dog had been given 3 mg/kg dexamethasone 2 days prior to the CBC. Glucocorticoids cause a mature neutrophilia by increasing release of mature neutrophils from the marrow storage pool, demarginating neutrophils from the marginal neutrophil pool (MNP) into the circulating neutrophil pool (CNP), and decreasing neutrophil migration into tissues. The leukocyte changes will revert to normal within a few days after cessation of glucocorticoid therapy. It is important that this leukocyte pattern not be confused with the response seen with inflammation.

This leukocyte pattern also can be typical of hyperadrenocorticism.

# NOTES

# CASE 3 Canine 15 Year Old Castrated Male Cocker Spaniel

**History** Vomiting for 5 days.

**Physical Examination** Dog is obese, depressed, and severely dehydrated.

## Laboratory Date

|  | Patient | Reference Range |  | Patient | Reference Range |
|---|---|---|---|---|---|
| PCV % | 42 | (37-55) | WBC/ul | 22,400 | (6,000-17,000) |
| Hgb g/dl | 14.0 | (12-18) | Neutrophils | 13,884 | (3,000-11,400) |
| RBC x10⁶/ul | 6.2 | (5.5-8.5) | Band cells | 2,240 | (0-300) |
| MCV fl | 67 | (60-77) | Lymphocytes | 1,568 | (1,000-4,800) |
| MCH pg | 22 | (19-24) | Monocytes | 4,256 | (150-1,350) |
| MCHC g/dl | 34 | (32-36) | Eosinophils | 224 | (100-750) |
| TPP g/dl | 9.0 | (6.0-7.5) |  |  |  |
| Platelets | ADQ |  |  |  |  |

Toxic neutrophils 3+

## Discussion/Interpretation

History of vomiting suggests that hyperproteinemia is due to dehydration. A leukocytosis is present due to a neutrophilia with a left shift (Figure C3-1) and monocytosis. Toxic change is evident in circulating neutrophils. The leukocyte pattern indicates acute inflammation with tissue necrosis. An abdominocentesis revealed a septic neutrophilic exudate (Figure C3-2). Serum amylase and lipase activities were both increased. The clinical diagnosis was necrotizing pancreatitis with septic peritonitis.

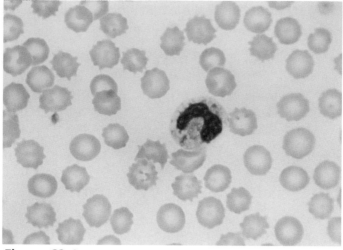

## Figure C3-1

Canine toxic band neutrophil. Inflammation or toxemia causes morphologic changes in neutrophils. In this band neutrophil, cytoplasmic basophilia, vacuolation, and a Dohle body are evident (100x).

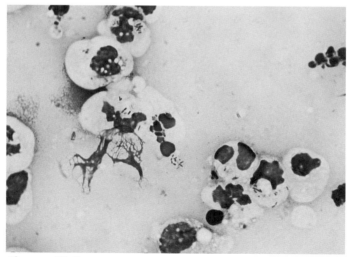

## Figure C3-2

Abdominal fluid. Swollen degenerate neutrophils with phagocytosed bacteria indicate septic peritonitis which has caused a left shift with toxic neutrophils in the CBC (100x).

# NOTES

# NOTES

# CASE 4  Canine 5 Year Old Spayed Female Sheepdog

**History**  Partial anorexia and intermittent vomiting. Owner reports that dog is "not her usual self" during the last 2 weeks.

**Physical Examination**  No abnormalities detected.

**Laboratory Date**

| | Patient | Reference Range | | Patient | Reference Range |
|---|---|---|---|---|---|
| PCV % | 35 | (37-55) | WBC/ul | 23,400 | (6,000-17,000) |
| Hgb g/dl | 11.9 | (12-18) | Neutrophils | 20,124 | (3,000-11,400) |
| RBC x10⁶/ul | 5.6 | (5.5-8.5) | Band cells | 234 | (0-300) |
| MCV fl | 66 | (60-77) | Lymphocytes | 1,404 | 1,000-4,800) |
| MCH pg | 22 | (19-24) | Monocytes | 1,638 | (150-1,350) |
| MCHC g/dl | 33 | (32-36) | Eosinophils | --- | (100-750) |
| TPP g/dl | 7.3 | (6.0-7.5) | | | |
| Plasma color | Normal | | | | |
| Reticulocytes % | 0.4 | (<1.0) | | | |
| Absolute Retic/ul | 22,400 | (<80,000) | | | |
| Platelets/uL | 231,000 | (>200,000) | | | |
| NRBC | 69/100WBC | | | | |

**RBC morphology**
Anisocytosis 1+
Target cells 2+
Basophilic stippling 1+

**Discussion/Interpretation**

The CBC is unusual in that there is mild anemia with numerous NRBCs (metarubricytes). However, the metarubricytosis is not accompanied by significant anisocytosis, macrocytosis, polychromasia, or an increase in reticulocytes (Figure C4-1). In addition, the anemia is mild and the number of NRBCs is out of proportion to the severity of anemia. This is a nonregenerative anemia because the response is disordered and causes of inappropriate metarubricytosis should be pursued. These include marrow neoplasia, myelofibrosis, lead poisoning, myelophthisis, extramedullary hematopoiesis, or severe anoxia. Basophilic stippling can be associated with lead poisoning but is not a consistent feature (Figure C4-2). Basophilic stippling can also be seen in blood films of dogs and cats with intense erythrogenic responses to severe anemia. In this dog, the inappropriate release of metarubricytes and the stippling are reasons to submit blood for lead analysis. The blood lead level was 1.6 ppm (normal Pb <0.35 ppm). A neutrophilic leukocytosis and monocytosis are present suggesting an inflammatory response with tissue necrosis.

**Diagnosis** Inappropriate metarubricytosis due to lead poisoning.

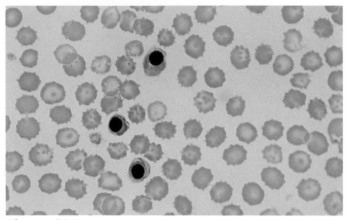

**Figure C4-1**
Canine blood. Several NRBCs are noted in the field that are not accompanied by polychromasia or anisocytosis. In a dog that has a very mild anemia, the NRBCs represent an inappropriate response. Causes of inappropriate metarubricytosis include acute anoxia, marrow neoplasia, myelofibrosis, extramedullary hematopoiesis, myelophthisis and lead poisoning (40x).

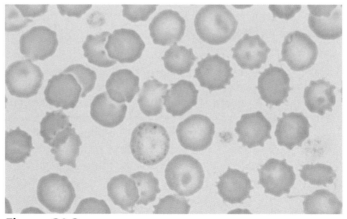

**Figure C4-2**
Canine blood. RBCs are crenated and several target cells are noted. Basophilic stippling is evident in the large RBC in center of the field as blue-black granules in the periphery of the cytoplasm. Basophilic stippling is an inconsistent finding in lead poisoning (120x).

# NOTES

# NOTES

# CASE 5   Feline 4 Year Old Castrated Male Domestic Longhair

**History**  Weight loss, anorexia, and listless for 3 weeks. Owner reports that cat never goes outside.

**Physical Examination**  Mucous membranes are white, rapid pulse, moderate weight loss, enlarged spleen and liver.

| | Patient | Reference Range | | Patient | Reference Range |
|---|---|---|---|---|---|
| PCV % | 12 | (30-40) | WBC/ul | 13,000 | 5,500-19,500) |
| Hgb g/dl | 4.2 | (8.5-15) | Neutrophils | 3,510 | (2,500-12,500) |
| RBC x10⁶/ul | 2.05 | (5.2-10) | Band cells | --- | (0-300) |
| MCV fl | 58 | (39-55) | Lymphocytes | 5,460 | (1,500-7,000) |
| MCH pg | 19 | (13-17) | Monocytes | 910 | (0-850) |
| MCHC g/dl | 35 | (30-36) | Eosinophils | 130 | (0-750) |

| | | |
|---|---|---|
| TPP g/dl | 7.7 | (6.0-7.5) |
| Platelets/ul | 170,000 | (>300,000) |
| Reticulocytes % | 1.0 | (<0.6%) |
| Absolute Retic/ul | 20,500 | (<80,000) |
| Plasma color | normal | |
| Blasts | 2,990 | |
| NRBC | 425/100WBC | |

**RBC Morphology:**
    Normal

**Discussion/Interpretation**

The uncorrected WBC count was 77,200/ul. The difference between this value and the reported WBC count is due to the correction for NRBCs. Severe anemia is present with an increase in MCV and numerous NRBCs. However, the increased MCV and metarubricytosis are not accompanied by anisocytosis, polychromasia, or reticulocytosis (Figure C5-1). The anemia in this cat is nonregenerative because the morphologic response was not orderly or proportional to the severity of anemia. Blast cells were quite large and had dark blue cytoplasm, focal perinuclear clear zone, round eccentric nucleus, and a single large nucleolus (Figures C5-2 and C5-3). Mitotic figures were noted occasionally. The presence of blast cells, nonregenerative anemia, and thrombocytopenia are indications for bone marrow examination. The increase in MCV is probably due to macrocytosis and the fact that the electronic counter is including large leukocytes and blast cells in the RBC volume analysis. FeLV antigen test was positive. A bone marrow aspirate revealed diffuse infiltration with blast cells identical to those seen in blood (Figure C5-4). Developing granulocytes and megakaryocytes were infrequent.

**Diagnosis**  Myeloproliferative neoplasm (Erythroleukemia)

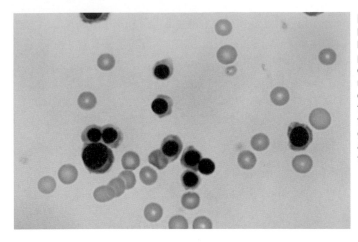

**Figure C5-1**
Feline blood. Numerous NRBCs are present without any evidence of polychromasia, macrocytosis, or anisocytosis. These findings indicate that the anemia is nonregenerative. Platelets are not observed in the field (100x).

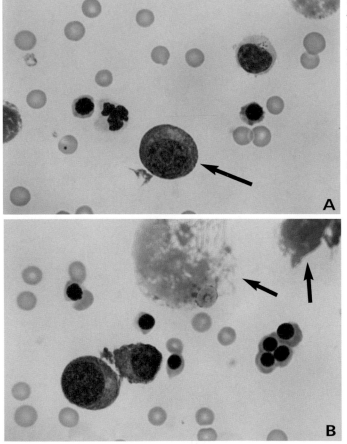

**Figure C5-2**
**A.** Blast cells (arrow) are noted that are larger than a neutrophil and have an eccentric nucleus, irregular chromatin, prominent nucleoli, and focal clear zone in a dark basophilic cytoplasm. **B.** Large amorphous pink staining aggregates (arrows) are disintegrated nuclei (100x).

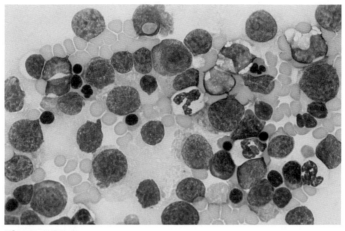

## Figure C5-3
Peripheral edge of smear. Numerous disintegrated nuclei of blast cells are concentrated on the feather edge of the smear. Blast cells are fragile and tend to fragment during the preparation of smears (100x).

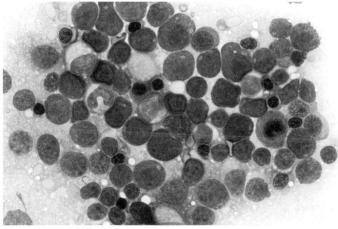

## Figure C5-4
Bone marrow. Nonregenerative anemia, NRBCs without poly-chromasia, and blast cells are clear indications for bone marrow examination. Normal granulocytic and erythroid cells have been replaced by a homogenous population of blast cells identical to those seen in blood. Because of this neoplastic proliferation, the cat is severely anemic, thrombocytopenic, and leukopenic (100x).

# NOTES

# CASE 6  Canine 11 Year Old Female Husky

**History**  Weight loss, diminished appetite, decreased exercise tolerance, loose stools for several weeks.

**Physical Examination**  Pale mucous membranes, dark tarry stools. Dog is fractious and difficult to examine.

| | Patient | Reference Range | | Patient | Reference Range |
|---|---|---|---|---|---|
| PCV % | 11 | (37-55) | WBC/ul | 27,400 | (6,000-17,000) |
| Hgb g/dl | 2.9 | (12-15) | Neutrophils | 19,454 | (3,000-11,400) |
| RBC x10⁶/ul | 2.66 | (5.5-8.5) | Band cells | ---- | (0-300) |
| MCV fl | 42 | (60-77) | Lymphocytes | 6,302 | (1,000-4,800) |
| MCH pg | 10 | (19-24) | Monocytes | 1,370 | (150-1,350) |
| MCHC g/dl | 23 | (32-36) | Eosinophils | 274 | (100-750) |

| | | |
|---|---|---|
| TPP g/dl | 6.0 | (6.0-7.5) |
| Plasma color | Normal | |
| Reticulocytes % | 3.3 | (<1.0) |
| Absolute Retic/ul | 87,780 | (<80,000) |
| Platelets/uL | 780,000 | (>200,000) |
| NRBC | 7/100WBC | |

**RBC morphology:**
   Anisocytosis 2+
   Microcytosis 2+
   Polychromasia 1+
   Hypochromia 3+
   Poikilocytosis 3+

## Discussion/Interpretation

Severe anemia and hypoproteinemia are evident. On initial inspection, it appears there is a regenerative response because of the anisocytosis, polychromasia, NRBCs, and reticulocyte increase. Several findings indicate that the regenerative response is abnormal. The RBC indices and morphology reveal a microcytic and hypochromic anemia (Figure C6-1) instead of the normal regenerative response to blood loss, which is macrocytic and hypochromic. Although the reticulocyte percentage is increased slightly, the absolute reticulocyte count does not indicate a significant reticulocyte response. Serum iron and serum iron binding capacity were measured and confirmed iron deficiency (Iron = 38 ug/dl,  Reference Range 89-138; IBC = 360 ug/dl, Reference Range 177-400). Although the change can be subtle, RBCs in iron deficient animals are smaller and have a much larger area of central pallor due to insufficient hemoglobin content (Figure C6-2). Polychromatophilic RBCs and NRBCs are poorly hemoglobinated and have a vacuolated or moth-eaten cytoplasms. Marked poikilocytosis and thrombocytosis are also features of iron deficiency. A mature neutrophilia, monocytosis, and lymphocytosis are evident in the leukogram and are consistent with chronic inflammation. A new steady state in neutrophil kinetics has evolved characterized by increased neutrophil production in marrow that is equal to tissue demand. Atypical lymphocytes or lymphoblasts were not observed on the blood film. The dog was sedated for a more thorough examination which revealed a firm mid-abdominal mass. Ultrasound examination confirmed an intestinal mass with mixed echogenicity. Fine needle aspiration of the abdominal mass revealed a pleomorphic population of epithelial cells (Figure C6-3).

**Diagnosis** Intestinal carcinoma (Figure C6-4) with chronic GI hemorrhage that caused a secondary iron deficiency anemia.

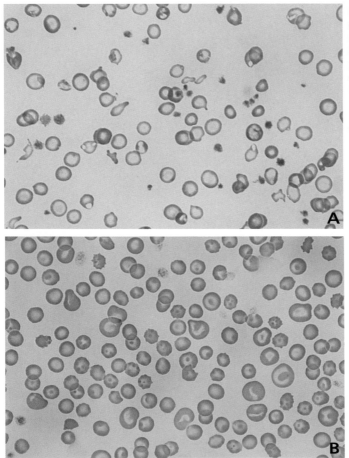

**Figure C6-1**
Canine blood. Blood from the dog in Case 6 is compared with normal canine RBCs. **A.** Microcytosis and hypochromia is pronounced when compared with the normal RBCs in **B** (40x).

### Figure C6-2

Canine blood. Microcytes, poikilocytes, and hypochromic RBCs are evident. Hypochromic RBCs have a larger area of central pallor with a thin and reduced rim of hemoglobin staining. Iron deficiency anemia is the most frequent cause of these changes in dogs and cats (100x).

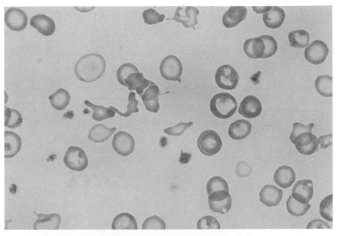

### Figure C6-3

Aspirate of abdominal mass. A sheet of pleomorphic epithelial cells with marked anisocytosis, anisokaryosis, variable N:C ratios, and irregular chromatin confirms the presence of carcinoma (100x).

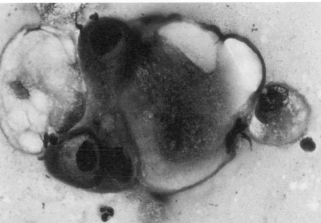

### Figure C6-4

Loop of bowel with large carcinoma. Note the ulcerated luminal surface which caused chronic hemorrhage and secondary iron deficiency anemia.

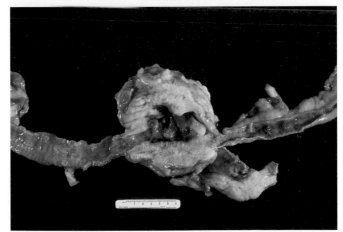

# NOTES

## CASE 7  Canine 4 Week Old Male Greyhound

**History**  Puppy was healthy at birth and during the first week of life. At 2-3 weeks of age, puppy became acutely depressed, stopped eating, and seemed pale. In spite of supportive care, about 50-60% of puppies in previous litters died within a few days of showing clinical signs.

**Physical Examination**  Moderate depression, weakness, lack of appetite, fever (T= 103.8°F) and mucous membranes are pale and icteric. Feces are formed and bright orange in color. The spleen is enlarged. The puppy is heavily infested with ticks.

| | Patient | Reference Range | | Patient | Reference Range |
|---|---|---|---|---|---|
| PCV % | 10% | (37-55) | WBC/ul | 33,000 | (6,000-17,000) |
| Hgb g/dl | 2.9 | (12-18) | Neutrophils | 27,000 | (3,000-11,400) |
| RBC x10⁶/ul | 1.43 | (4.95-7.87) | Band cells | 3,500 | (0-300) |
| MCV fl | 70 | (60-77) | Lymphocytes | 800 | (1,000-4,800) |
| MCH pg | 20 | (19-24) | Monocytes | 1,700 | (150-1,350) |
| MCHC g/dl | 29 | (32-36) | Eosinophils | ---- | (100-750) |

| | Patient | Reference Range |
|---|---|---|
| TPP g/dl | 4.5 | (6.0-7.5) |
| Reticulocytes % | 10.2 | (<1.0) |
| Absolute Retic/ul | 145,800 | (<80,000) |
| Plasma color | 4+icterus | |
| Platelets/ul | 35,000 | (>200,000) |

### RBC Morphology
Anisocytosis 3+
Polychromasia 3+
Macrocytosis 3+

| Selected Chemistries | Patient | Reference Range |
|---|---|---|
| Alanine Aminotransferase (ALT) IU/L | 156 | (4-66) |
| Total Bilirubin mg/dl | 12.4 | (0.1-0.6) |

### Urine
| | |
|---|---|
| Color | Amber |
| SG | 1.035 |
| pH | 6 |
| Bilirubin | 4+ |
| Blood | 1+ |
| Protein | 1+ |
| Sediment | Bile crystals |

### Fecal flotation
Few hookworm ova

## Discussion/Interpretation

The RBC morphology and reticulocytosis indicate regenerative anemia. Icterus, bilirubinuria, splenomegaly, and orange colored feces and the absence of hemorrhage indicate hemolytic disease. Causes of hemolysis include infectious agents, toxins, immune-mediated destruction, fragmentation, osmotic lysis, and congenital hemolytic disease. The blood films were reexamined for the presence of RBC parasites, Heinz bodies, spherocytes, schistocytes, and ghosts. Serologic tests for Leptospira were negative. A direct Coombs' test was positive. A few *Babesia canis* organisms were identified in RBCs on the initial blood film (Figure C7-1). Impression smear of spleen from a dead puppy revealed numerous Babesia organisms within RBCs (Figure C7-2). Puppies were treated with diminazene aceturate. Aggressive tick control was initiated to control the transmission via ticks.

The absence of an increase in MCV and the hypoproteinemia are likely due to blood loss and iron depletion secondary to hookworm disease. Hemolytic anemia and thrombocytopenia in Babesiosis are caused by immune-mediated destruction that targets RBCs and platelets. Thus, it is not unusual for the Coombs' test to be positive.

White cell data indicate an inflammatory leukogram with superimposed stress and tissue necrosis. Such a pattern is common in hemolytic conditions. The cause of the inflammatory response is the destruction of circulating red cells.

## Diagnosis

Hemolytic anemia due to *Babesia canis* complicated by hookworm disease.

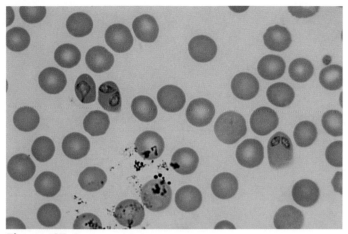

**Figure C7-1**
*Babesia canis*. Pairs of basophilic, pyriform, protozoal organisms are noted in the RBCs. Stain precipitate is also present as basophilic granules covering some RBCs (100x).

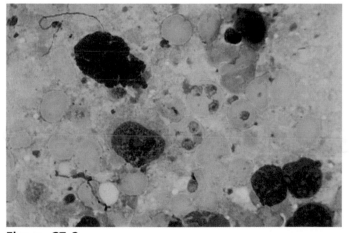

**Figure C7-2**
Splenic impression smear, *Babesia canis*. Round to oval parasites are noted within several RBCs. Round basophilic nuclear structure is noted within each protozoal organism. Disintegrated nuclei of lymphocytes are noted as round pink amorphous aggregates (100x).

# NOTES

# CASE 8  Canine 5 Year Old Female Cocker Spaniel

**History**  Owner states that dog is not well and that urine appears very dark. Treated with antibiotics for a bladder infection by the previous veterinarian.

**Physical Examination**  T=104°F, mucous membranes are pale and icteric, large firm mass in mid-abdomen. Mild dehydration is present.

| | Patient | Reference Range | | Patient | Reference Range |
|---|---|---|---|---|---|
| PCV % | 11.5 | (37-55) | WBC/ul | 46,000 | (6,000-17,000) |
| Hgb g/dl | 3.4 | (12-18) | Neutrophils | 34,120 | (3,000-11,400) |
| RBC x10⁶/ul | 1.3 | (4.95-7.87) | Band cells | 3,600 | (0-300) |
| MCV fl | 88 | (60-77) | Lymphocytes | 2,300 | (1,000-4,800) |
| MCH pg | 26 | (19-24) | Monocytes | 3,680 | (150-1,350) |
| MCHC g/dl | 29 | (32-36) | Eosinophils | 460 | (100-750) |

| | | |
|---|---|---|
| TPP g/dl | 8.3 | (6.0-7.5) |
| Plasma color | Icteric, slight hemolysis | |
| Reticulocytes % | 23 | (<1.0) |
| Absolute Retic/ul | 299,000 | (<80,000) |
| Platelets/ul | 240,000 | (>200,000) |

NRBC     1,840/100WBC

**RBC Morphology**
Anisocytosis, macrocytosis, polychromasia 3+
Spherocytes 3+
Ghosts 1+
Agglutination 1+

| Selected Chemistries | Patient | Reference Range |
|---|---|---|
| Total Bilirubin | 7.9 mg/dl | (0.1-0.6) |
| ALT | 693 IU/L | (4-66) |

## Discussion/Interpretation

The clinical presentation and laboratory data could lead in several different directions. Icterus, increased total bilirubin and increased ALT activity could indicate liver disease. Abdominal mass, fever, neutrophilic leukocytosis, left shift and monocytosis are compatible with inflammatory disease such as pyometra in an intact female.

Icterus can be caused by hemolytic disease, hepatic disease, or bile duct obstruction. In an icteric animal, always check first for evidence of hemolytic anemia. The CBC results indicate a marked regenerative response (increased reticulocytes and MCV) and the slide examination reveals anisocytosis, polychromasia, macrocytosis, NRBCs, and numerous spherocytes and ghosts (Figures C8-1, C8-2, C8-3, and C8-4). These findings are consistent with hemolytic anemia due to immune-mediated RBC destruction. No RBC parasites were observed. The increased total protein is likely due to dehydration.

The leukocytosis with left shift is very pronounced but can be a feature of immune-mediated hemolytic anemia. The increases in ALT and total bilirubin represent the combined effects of acute RBC destruction with excess bilirubin production and secondary liver damage due to hypoxic injury as a result of severe acute anemia.

**Diagnosis** Immune-mediated hemolytic disease, Coombs' positive.

**Outcome** Responded to prednisone therapy.

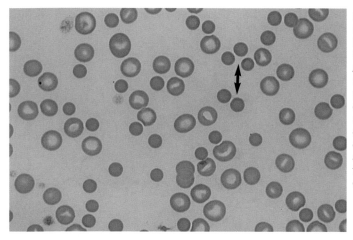

**Figure C8-1**
RBCs from dog with immune-mediated hemolytic anemia. Anisocytosis is marked due to the presence of macrocytic polychromatophilic erythrocytes and spherocytes (arrow) which are the smaller cells that lack the normal central pallor. (60x)

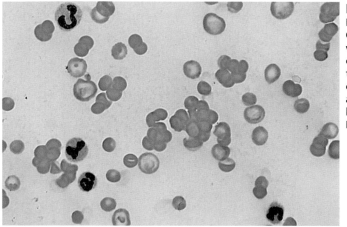

**Figure C8-2**
RBC agglutination. Clustering of RBCs in variable groups indicates that agglutination is present. This change is caused by antibody bridging between adjacent RBCs. (60x)

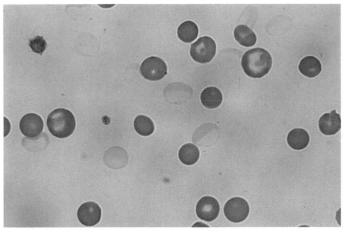

### Figure C8-3
Spherocytes and ghost RBCs are present. The latter indicate some degree of intravascular lysis (100x).

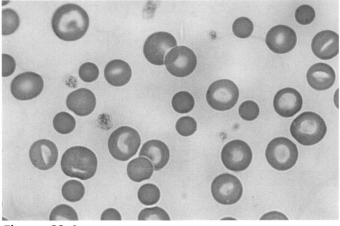

### Figure C8-4
Marked regenerative response is evidenced by marked anisocytosis, macrocytosis, and polychromasia. Smaller RBCs without central pallor are spherocytes.

# NOTES

# CASE 9 Canine 2 Year Old Intact Female Labrador

**History** Forelimb lameness, fever and loss of appetite for 3 weeks. Dog was treated with antibiotics for 2 weeks with no improvement.

**Clinical signs** T 105°F, pain in right humerus, cough with moist rales, enlarged peripheral lymph nodes. No evidence of dehydration.

|  | Patient | Reference Range |  | Patient | Reference Range |
|---|---|---|---|---|---|
| PCV % | 30 | (37-55) | WBC/ul | 46,300 | 6000-17,000) |
| Hgb g/dl | 10.2 | (12-15) | Neutrophils | 42,133 | (3,000-11,400) |
| RBC x10⁶/ul | 4.3 | (5.5-8.5) | Band cells | 926 | (0-300) |
| MCV fl | 70 | (60-77) | Lymphocytes | 926 | (1,000-4,800) |
| MCH pg | 23 | (19-24) | Monocytes | 1,852 | (150-1,350) |
| MCHC g/dl | 34 | (32-36) | Eosinophils | 463 | (100-750) |
| TPP g/dl | 8.8 | 6.0-7.5) | | | |
| Plasma color | Normal | | | | |
| Reticulocytes % | 0.9 | (<1.0) | | | |
| Absolute Retic/ul | 38,700 | (<80,000) | | | |
| Platelets | ADQ | | | | |

**RBC morphology**
Normal

### Discussion/Interpretation

Mild anemia is evident with increased total protein concentration. Anemia is normocytic and normochromic (Figure C9-1). Physical examination reveals no evidence of hemorrhage. Reticulocyte count and RBC morphology indicate no evidence of regeneration, which should be expected with hemorrhage or hemolysis and a 3 week history of disease. The increase in total protein can be due to dehydration or increased globulin synthesis in response to infection/inflammation. Since there is no evidence of dehydration, hyperglobulinemia is the likely cause. The WBC count is increased due to a moderate to marked neutrophilia with a monocytosis and a minimal left shift (2% of the WBCs in the differential count are band neutrophils). These findings are consistent with chronic inflammation. The decrease in lymphocyte numbers is due to endogenous glucocorticoid release or stress response.

The bone marrow was cellular with an increased myeloid:erythroid (M:E) ratio (Figure C9-2). Granulopoiesis was active with normal maturation. Erythroid precursors were reduced in number but maturation appeared normal. Marrow iron stores were increased.

**Summary**  Nonregenerative anemia, hyperglobulinemia, and neutrophilic leukocytosis with minimal left shift and monocytosis. Bone marrow has increased iron stores and a predominance of granulocytic cells with a reduction in erythroid precursors indicating granulocytic hyperplasia and erythroid hypoplasia. These findings are consistent with anemia of inflammation.

**Outcome**  Fine needle aspirate of lymph nodes and lung reveal pyogranulomatous inflammation due *Blastomyces dermatitidis* (Figure C9-3).

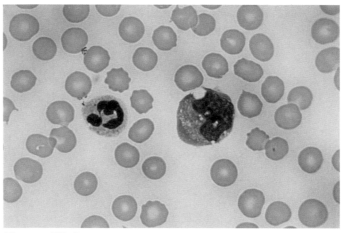

**Figure C9-1**
Canine blood. Normocytic, normochromic RBCs indicate that the anemia is nonregenerative. Segmented neutrophil and monocyte are in the field. Neutrophilia and monocytosis indicated chronic inflammation with tissue necrosis (100x).

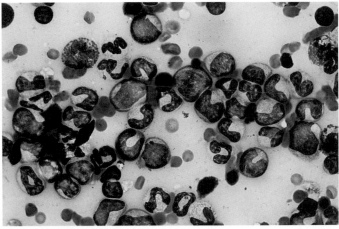

### Figure C9-2
Bone marrow. Granulocytic hyperplasia and erythroid hypoplasia are evident in the marrow smear. The majority of cells are developing granulocytes with a marked reduction in erythroid activity. The CBC and marrow changes are consistent with chronic inflammation (40x).

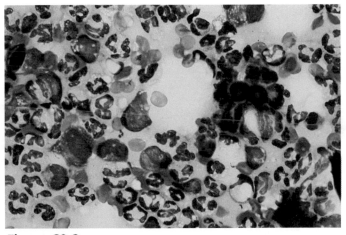

### Figure C9-3
Aspirate of lymph node. Pyogranulomatous inflammation is present in the node. Majority of cells are neutrophils and macrophages with a broad-based budding yeast visible to the right of center. Morphology of yeast is consistent with *Blastomyces dermatitidis*.

# NOTES

# CASE 10   9 Year Old Neutered Male Gordon Setter

**History**  Adopted from humane society 1 year ago.  Owner has noticed increased hair shedding and decreased physical activity.

**Physical Examination**  Normal body temperature.  Increased pulse rate. Bilaterally symmetrical alopecia with severe weakness, weight loss, and pale mucous membranes.  Abdominal mass detected on abdominal palpation.

|  | Patient | Reference Range |  | Patient | Reference Range |
|---|---|---|---|---|---|
| PCV % | 9 | (37-55) | WBC/ul | 3,895 | (6,000-17,000) |
| Hgb g/dl | 3.0 | (12-15) | Neutrophils | 2,804 | (3,000-11,400) |
| RBC x10⁶/ul | 1.3 | (5.5-8.5) | Band cells | --- | (0-300) |
| MCV fl | 69 | (60-77) | Lymphocytes | 1,051 | (1,000-4,800) |
| MCH pg | 23 | (19-24) | Monocytes | 39 | (150-1,350) |
| MCHC g/dl | 33 | (32-36) | Eosinophils | --- | (100-750) |
| TPP g/dl | 7.1 | (6.0-7.5) |  |  |  |
| Plasma color | Normal |  |  |  |  |
| Reticulocytes % | 0.8 | (<1.0) |  |  |  |
| Absolute Retic/ul | 10,400 | (<80,000) |  |  |  |
| Platelets/ul | 43,000 | (>200,000) |  |  |  |

**RBC morphology**
  No abnormalities

## Discussion/Interpretation

A severe anemia is present with normal RBC indices and no evidence of regeneration in the RBC morphology or reticulocyte count (Figure C10-1).  Severe thrombocytopenia, leukopenia, and neutropenia are present.  These findings indicate a severe decrease in circulating blood cells or pancytopenia.  Bone marrow aspiration is indicated.

Bone marrow examination revealed a severely hypocellular marrow with very few erythroid, granulocytic, or megakaryocytic precursors (Figure C10-2).  An occasional capillary fragment is noted.  Most of the marrow has been replaced with fat tissue.

**Diagnosis**  Severe pancytopenia due to marrow hypoplasia/destruction. Consider toxic chemicals, drugs, infectious agents, or immune-mediated disease as possible causes.

**Outcome**  Ultrasound guided FNA of abdominal mass reveals a Sertoli cell tumor.  Metastasis is evident in the regional lymph nodes.  These tumors can secrete high levels of estrogen resulting in symmetrical alopecia and severe marrow hypoplasia.  Serum estrogen levels were measured and levels were extremely high. Because of metastatic disease in the iliac and sublumbar lymph nodes, the owner elected euthanasia. The owner subsequently discovered that the dog had not been neutered and was a bilateral cryptorchid.

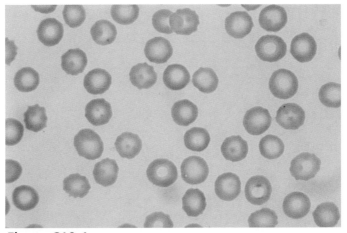

**Figure C10-1**
Canine blood. Severe nonregenerative anemia and thrombocytopenia are evident. Polychromasia, anisocytosis, and macrocytosis are absent. Platelets are rarely seen (100x).

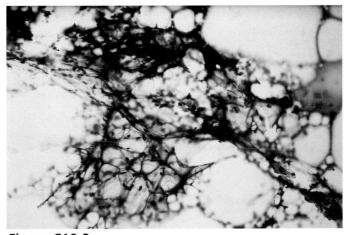

**Figure C10-2**
Bone marrow. Replacement of the normal marrow cells with adipose tissue and connective tissue indicates severe marrow hypoplasia. Reduction in marrow activity results in pancytopenia. This change can be caused by toxins, drugs, infectious agents, chemical injury, and immune-mediated disease.

# NOTES

# CASE 11  Feline 10 Month Old Female Siamese

**History**  Straining in an attempt to deliver kittens.

**Physical Examination**  T =104.9°F, depressed, dehydrated, serohemor-
rhagic vaginal discharge; radiographs reveal macerated fetuses in genital
tract.

|  | Day 1 | Patient Day 2 | Day 5 | Reference Range |
|---|---|---|---|---|
| PCV % | 46 | 38 | 29 | (30-40) |
| TPP g/dl | 7.0 | 4.6 | 4.5 | (6.0-7.5) |
| Platelets | ADQ | ADQ | ADQ | |
| WBC/ul | 9,500 | 9,100 | 48,400 | (5,500-19,500) |
| Neutrophils | 2,755 | 3,003 | 45,980 | (2,500-12,500) |
| Band cells | 5,415 | 4,914 | 1,452 | (0-300) |
| Metarubricytes | 95 | 273 | --- | |
| Lymphocytes | 665 | 637 | 484 | (1,500-7,000) |
| Monocytes | 570 | 273 | 484 | (0-850) |
| Eosinophils | --- | --- | --- | (0-750) |
| Toxic neutrophils | 3+ | 3+ | --- | |

## Discussion/Interpretation

Day 1

Polycythemia is due to dehydration. Normal TPP in light of severe
dehydration indicates hypoproteinemia. Leukogram reveals severe
degenerative left shift, lymphopenia, and toxic neutrophils (Figures
C11-1, 11-2, and 11-3). These changes are compatible with overwhelming or peracute inflammation of a well-vascularized tissue or
body cavity. The severity of the left shift (bands exceed mature neutrophils with a normal WBC count) indicates a poor prognosis. Acute
peritonitis or metritis is a likely cause. Hypoproteinemia is due to protein leakage associated with acute inflammation. Abdominocentesis
reveals a neutrophilic exudate with rod-shaped
bacteria (Figure C11-4).

Day 2

Cat was given IV fluids and antibiotics prior to exploratory laparotomy.
With rehydration, PCV is reduced to normal and the hypoproteinemia
is evident. Leukocyte values are similar to day 1 and indicate acute
overwhelming inflammation and sepsis. Severe lymphopenia on both
days is due to stress response. Exploratory surgery revealed acute
metritis with a uterine perforation resulting in acute diffuse peritonitis.
Ovariohystorectomy and abdominal lavage were done.

Day 5

CBC is 2 days postoperative and reveals a marked neutrophilic leuko-cytosis with left shift and severe lymphopenia. The leukocyte response from day 2 to day 4 is caused by the abrupt removal of the site of inflammation. A rebound neutrophilia occurs because of continued production and release of neutrophils from a stimulated bone marrow. Hypoproteinemia persists and will recover gradually during the next 2 weeks. PCV is reduced due to blood loss at surgery and the presence of severe inflammation.

**Outcome** Uneventful recovery

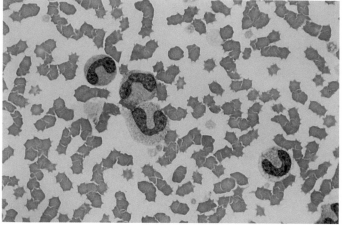

**Figure C11-1**
Feline blood. Increase in band neutrophils indicates a severe left shift. Increased rouleaux formation can be caused by changes in plasma proteins as a result of inflam-mation (40x).

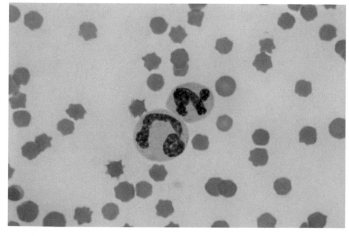

**Figure C11-2**
Feline blood. Inflammation can produce changes in neutrophil morphol-ogy. Two segmented neutrophils are pres-ent that have a slight increase in cytoplasmic basophilia. One of the neutrophils is very large and has abnormal nuclear lobulation which is a sign of toxic change (100x).

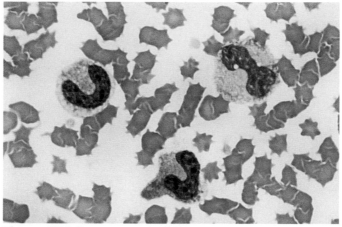

**Figure C11-3**
Feline blood. RBCs are crenated with marked rouleaux formation. Band neutrophils are extremely toxic with basophilic granular cytoplasm and Dohle bodies (100x).

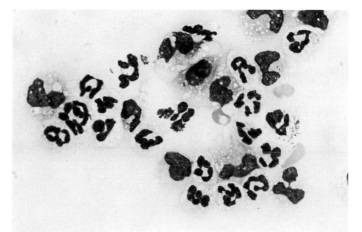

**Figure C11-4**
Abdominal fluid. Mixture of neutrophils and macrophages are present. Phagocytosed bacteria are noted. These findings confirm septic peritonitis (100x).

# NOTES

# CASE 12  Canine 1 Year Old Intact Male Collie

**History**  Severe vomiting and diarrhea for 12 hours.

**Physical Examination**  T= 98°F, P 40, 8% dehydration; dog is very weak and nearly comatose.

| | Patient | Reference Range | | Patient | Reference Range |
|---|---|---|---|---|---|
| PCV % | 60 | (37-55) | WBC/ul | 11,300 | (6,000-17,000) |
| Hgb g/dl | 20.5 | (12-15) | Neutrophils | 8,136 | (3,000-11,400) |
| RBC x10⁶/ul | 8.9 | (5.5-8.5) | Band cells | 113 | (0-300) |
| MCV fl | 67 | (60-77) | Lymphocytes | 1,928 | (1,000-4,800) |
| MCH pg | 23 | (19-24) | Monocytes | 678 | (150-1,350) |
| MCHC g/dl | 34 | (32-36) | Eosinophils | 452 | (100-750) |
| TPP g/dl | 9.3 | (6.0-7.5) | | | |
| Platelets | ADQ | | | | |

## Discussion/Interpretation

Polycythemia and hyperproteinemia are due to dehydration. The leukogram reveals a normal neutrophil and lymphocyte count. The leukocyte response is not indicative of inflammation or sepsis that would be significant considerations in the differential diagnosis. With the severity of clinical signs, we would expect at least a stress leukogram. A normal leukogram with these clinical signs is indicative of diminished levels of adrenal steroids that are characteristic of acute adrenocortical insufficiency (Addison's disease).

Serum chemistries revealed prerenal azotemia, hyponatremia, hyperkalemia, and a low baseline cortisol followed by a minimal response to ACTH stimulation.

# NOTES

# CASE 13   Canine 1 Year Old Intact Female Boxer

**History**  Hit by car 2 days prior to admission. Owner noticed that dog was not eating and was depressed.

**Physical examination**  Multiple abrasions. Area of pain over entire left side of abdomen.

|  | Patient | | | Reference Range |
|---|---|---|---|---|
|  | Day 1 | Day 2 (AM) | Day 2 (PM) |  |
| PCV % | 39 | 36 | 39 | (37-55) |
| TPP g/dl | 6.8 | 7.3 | 7.0 | (6.0-7.5) |
| Platelets | ADQ | ADQ | Decreased |  |
| WBC/ul | 19,500 | 13,600 | 3,800 | (6,000-17,000) |
| Neutrophils | 17,355 | 11,520 | 1,178 | (3,000-11,400) |
| Band cells | --- | 1,360 | 1,216 | (0-300) |
| Lymphocytes | 390 | 680 | 912 | (1,000-4,800) |
| Monocytes | 780 | 408 | 494 | (150-1,350) |
| Eosinophils | 975 | --- | --- | (100-750) |
| Toxic neutrophils | ---- | 2+ | 3+ |  |

**Abdominal Fluid (Day 2)**
  Color: cloudy, red tinged
  TP: 4.7 g/dl
  WBC: 23,000/ul
  Diff: 93% neutrophils

## Discussion/Interpretation

Day 1

A neutrophilic leukocytosis and lymphopenia are present. Toxic neutrophils or a left shift were not observed. These findings are consistent with a stress response. However, an early (mild) inflammatory response cannot be ruled out.

Day 2 (8AM)

The condition of the dog has deteriorated clinically. Depression, poor capillary refill time, and a rapid pulse are evident. The number of leukocytes and neutrophils has decreased and there is a marked left shift with toxic neutrophils (Figure C13-1). Acute inflammation or sepsis is likely. A careful search for site or organ system involved should be undertaken. Abdominocentesis revealed a septic neutrophilic exudate indicating acute peritonitis (Figure C13-2).

Day 2 (3PM)

Diffuse peritonitis was evident on surgical exploration. Multiple segments of infarcted bowel were resected. A CBC just prior to surgery revealed a marked reduction in neutrophil numbers with a severe degenerative left shift and toxic neutrophils. This change occurred over a 7-hour period and is indicative of severe overwhelming inflammation and a very grave prognosis. The decrease in platelets is likely due to consumption at sites of thrombosis and infarction. The dog died shortly after the surgery.

This case illustrates the dynamic and abrupt changes that can occur in the leukogram in response to acute overwhelming inflammation.

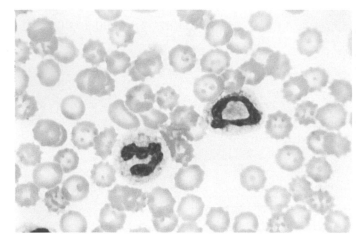

**Figure C13-1**
Canine blood. Both neutrophils exhibit toxic change in the form of cytoplasmic basophilia, vacuolation, and Dohle bodies. RBCs are crenated (100x).

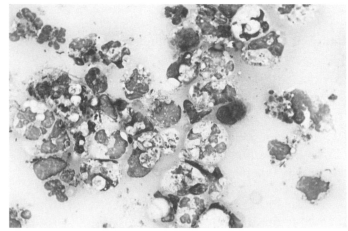

**Figure C13-2**
Abdominal fluid. Numerous degenerate neutrophils that contain a mixed population of phagocytosed bacteria are present in a proteinaceous background. Cytologic findings confirm septic peritonitis (100x).

# CASE 14   Feline 10 Year Old Castrated Male Tabby DSH

**History**   Episodes of vomiting and respiratory distress.  Respiratory signs are unresponsive to antibiotics.

**Physical Examination**   Normal body temperature with increased respiratory rate and expiratory effort.  Chest radiographs reveal several nodular radiopaque densities in the lungs.  Moderate dehydration is present.

| | Patient | Reference Range | | Patient | Reference Range |
|---|---|---|---|---|---|
| PCV% | 40 | (30-40) | WBC/ul | 17,000 | (5,500-19,500) |
| Hgb g/dl | 13.1 | (8.5-15) | Neutrophils | 6,120 | (2,500-12,500) |
| RBC x10⁶/ul | 8.6 | (5.2-10) | Band cells | --- | (0-300) |
| MCV fl | 46 | (39-55) | Lymphocytes | 2,040 | (1,500-7,000) |
| MCH pg | 15.2 | (13-17) | Monocytes | 340 | (0-850) |
| MCHC g/dl | 33 | (30-36) | Eosinophils | 8,500 | (0-750) |
| TPP g/dl | 8.6 | (6.0-7.5) | | | |

## Discussion/Interpretation

Increase in PCV and TPP is due to dehydration. Leukocytosis is due to a marked eosinophilia. Causes include allergy and hypersensitivity reactions, chronic granulomatous disease, and neoplasms such as mast cell tumors or lymphoma. Eosinophilic leukemia and hypereosinophilic syndrome are infrequent causes. Parasites that reside in the lung or that have a significant tissue migration phase or exposure to the immune response are frequent causes. Allergic or granulomatous diseases of the skin, respiratory tract, female genital tract or gastrointestinal tract are also likely to produce an eosinophilic leukocytosis. Because of the respiratory signs, *Paragonimus* (lung fluke), *Aleurostrongylus* (nematode), feline heartworm, and feline asthma were considered. A transtracheal wash revealed numerous eosinophils with a few macrophages (Figure C14-1). A few large, oval, rust-colored, operculated eggs (Figure C14-2) were also noted and confirm a diagnosis of *Paragonimus* infection.

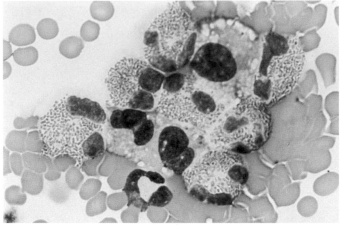

### Figure C14-1

Transtracheal wash. Numerous eosinophils are present in the transtracheal wash indicate allergy, hypersensitivity reaction, respiratory parasites, or possible heartworm infection (100x).

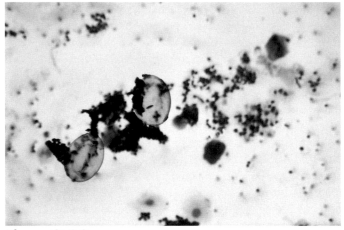

### Figure C14-2

Transtracheal wash. Low power scan of the sample reveals a few yellow oval *Paragonimus* eggs. The operculum on the eggs is not visible at this magnification. This lung fluke causes severe eosinophilic inflammation in the lung and airways (20x).

# NOTES

# NOTES

# CASE 15  Canine 14 Year Old Intact Female Cocker Spaniel

**History**  Dog was presented in a state of acute collapse. The dog resides in a household with numerous pets and prior history was vague.

**Physical Examination**  The animal is in fair body condition and has a purulent vaginal discharge. T = 98.7°F, rapid pulse, poor capillary refill time, moderate dehydration,and congested mucous membranes.

|  | Patient | | Reference Range |
|---|---|---|---|
|  | Day 1 | Day 3 | |
| PCV% | 38 | 31 | (37-55) |
| Hgb g/dl | 12.6 | 10.3 | (12-18) |
| RBC x10⁶/ul | 5.6 | 4.6 | (5.5-8.5) |
| MCV fl | 68 | 67 | (60-77) |
| MCH pg | 23 | 22 | (19-24) |
| MCHC g/dl | 33 | 34 | (32-36) |
| TPP | 6.7 | 5.2 | (6.0-7.5) |
| Platelets | ADQ | ADQ | |
| **RBC morphology** Normal | | | |
| WBC/uL | 7,700 | 21,800 | (6,000-17,000) |
| Neutrophils | 3,773 | 18,748 | (3,000-11,500) |
| Band cells | 2,233 | 436 | (0-300) |
| Metamyelocytes | 154 | 0 | |
| Lymphocytes | 1,155 | 654 | (1,000-4,800) |
| Monocytes | 308 | 1,962 | (150-1,350) |
| Toxic neutrophils | 2+ | --- | |

Abdominal paracentesis: exudate with degenerate neutrophils and rod-shaped bacteria.

**Discussion/Interpretation**

Day 1

The PCV and TPP are at the low end of normal and indicate anemia and hypoproteinemia when considered in light of moderate dehydration. The leukogram reveals a low normal WBC count with a severe left shift and toxic neutrophils. This response indicates acute overwhelming inflammation of a large, well-vascularized tissue or organ. The inflammation is severe enough to have depleted the marrow storage pool of mature and band neutrophils and initiate release of metamyelocytes. Causes of this type of response include acute peritonitis, necrotizing pancreatitis, acute suppurative pneumonia, acute cellulitis, or GI perforation. A poor prognosis is indicated because the WBC and segmented neutrophils counts are low, and band neutrophils exceed the number of segmented cells. The site of inflammation must be identified quickly and steps taken to initiate treatment.

Radiographs and abdominocentesis indicate acute septic peritonitis (Figure C15-1). Exploratory surgery revealed acute metritis with uterine perforation and peritonitis.

Day 3

With rehydration, anemia and hypoproteinemia are apparent. The anemia is likely due to inflammation and hemorrhage during surgery. Hemorrhage may also cause hypoproteinemia but leakage of plasma protein associated with diffuse inflammation is a factor in this case. A moderate leukocytosis with mild left shift and monocytosis is evident. Lymphopenia indicates stress. These changes are consistent with resolving inflammation and indicate that the bone marrow has repopulated the maturation pool of mature neutrophils and that the tissue demand for neutrophils has subsided. The prognosis is much improved.

**Outcome**  Recovery was uneventful. Reliance on total WBC counts alone in assessing the leukogram can be misleading. When the dog was in critical condition (Day 1) the total WBC count was normal. During recovery, the total WBC count was increased. However, the severe left shift and toxic neutrophils on Day 1 indicated the true magnitude and severity of disease.

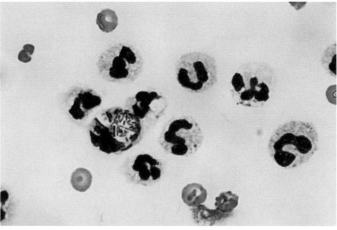

**Figure C15-1**
Abdominal fluid. Mixture of degenerate and nondegenerate neutrophils with phagocytosed rod-shaped bacteria indicates septic peritonitis (100x).

# NOTES

_____

_____

_____

_____

_____

_____

_____

_____

_____

_____

_____

_____

_____

_____

_____

_____

_____

_____

_____

_____

# NOTES

# CASE 16 Feline 9 Year Old Spayed Female Persian

**History** Cat has been treated with several drugs for respiratory and urinary tract infections.

**Physical Examination** The cat is depressed, listless, and has pale mucous membranes.

|  | Patient | Reference Range |  | Patient | Reference Range |
|---|---|---|---|---|---|
| PCV % | 13 | (30-40) | WBC/ul | 17,600 | (5,500-19,500) |
| Hgb g/dl | 4.2 | (8.5-15) | Neutrophils | 11,440 | (2,500-12,500) |
| RBC x10⁶/ul | 2.25 | (5.2-10) | Band cells | 176 | (0-300) |
| MCV fl | 57 | (39-55) | Lymphocytes | 4,752 | (1,500-7,000) |
| MCH pg | 19 | (13-17) | Monocytes | 1,232 | (0-850) |
| MCHC g/dl | 32 | (30-36) | Eosinophils | -- | (0-750) |
| TPP g/dl | 7.1 | (6.0-7.5) |  |  |  |
| Platelets/ul | 525,000 | (>300,000) |  |  |  |
| Reticulocytes % | 11 | (<0.6%) |  |  |  |
| Absolute Retic/ul | 247,500 | (<80,000) |  |  |  |
| Plasma color | Normal |  |  |  |  |
| NRBCs | 50/100WBC |  |  |  |  |

## RBC Morphology
Anisocytosis, Macrocytosis, Polychromasia 3+
Ghosts 1+
Howell Jolly bodies 2+
Heinz bodies 3+

## Discussion/Interpretation

The cat has a marked regenerative anemia as evidenced by increased MCV, anisocytosis, polychromasia, reticulocytosis, and increase in NRBCs (Figures C16-1 and C16-2). The normal TPP and physical examination eliminate hemorrhage as a cause. Hemolytic anemia can be caused by infectious agents such as RBC parasites, immune-mediated disease, fragmentation, osmotic lysis, and toxins. Heinz bodies indicate oxidative injury due to drugs, chemicals, plant sources, or metabolic disease (Figures C16-3 and C16-4). The presence of Heinz bodies will falsely elevate the hemoglobin measurement and cause increases in the MCH and MCHC. With the marked regenerative response, a decrease in MCHC is expected but the false increase in hemoglobin causes this value to remain within the reference range. Heinz bodies can be an incidental finding in the cat but when accompanied by marked regenerative anemia, the history should be re-examined for possible causes of Heinz body hemolysis. All previous medications were examined and one was found that contained methylene blue as part of its formulation. This compound is one of several that can cause Heinz body hemolytic anemia. Other drugs to consider include acetaminophen, benzocaine, DL methionine, phenazopyridine, and vitamin K3.

**Diagnosis** Drug-induced Heinz body hemolytic anemia

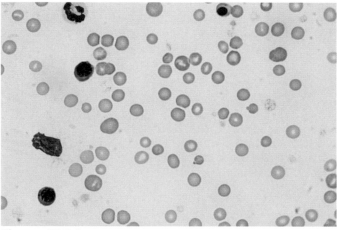

**Figure C16-1**
Feline blood. Anisocytosis, macrocytosis, polychromasia, and several NRBCs indicate regenerative anemia (40x).

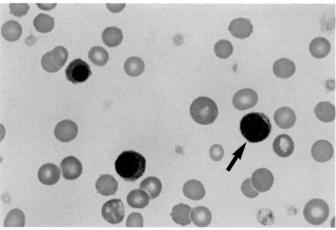

**Figure C16-2**
Feline blood. Two NRBCs are compared with a small lymphocyte (arrow). Platelet numbers are adequate and a few macrocytic polychromatophilic RBCs are present (100x).

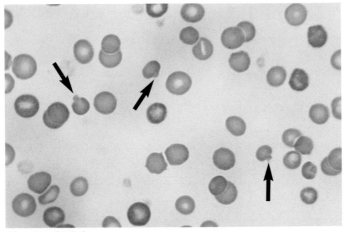

## Figure C16-3

Feline blood. Small rounded projections are noted on three RBCs (arrows). These inclusions are Heinz bodies which are caused by oxidative injury. The regenerative anemia in this case is due to hemolysis secondary to Heinz body formation (100x).

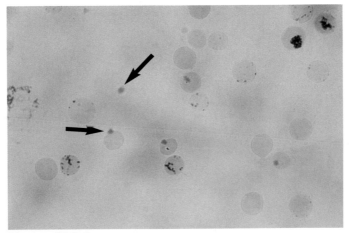

## Figure C16-4

Feline blood, reticulocyte stain. Reticulocytes are frequent. Both aggregate and punctate reticulocytes can be seen. Heinz bodies are small rounded turquoise inclusions (arrows) on the edge of the RBC membrane (100x).

# NOTES

# CASE 17 Feline 4 Year Old Intact Female DSH

**History** Anorexia, pendulous abdomen; owners believes cat is pregnant.

**Physical Examination** T=104.3°F cat is depressed, dehydrated, and has a serosanguinous vaginal discharge.

| | Patient | Reference Range | | Patient | Reference Range |
|---|---|---|---|---|---|
| PCV % | 28 | (30-40) | WBC/ul | 123,600 | (5,500-19,500) |
| Hgb g/dl | 9.9 | (8.5-15) | Neutrophils | 86,520 | (2,500-12,500) |
| RBC x10⁶/ul | 6.6 | (5.2-10) | Band cells | 22,248 | (0-300) |
| MCV fl | 42 | (39-55) | Metamyelocytes | 3,708 | (0) |
| MCH pg | 15 | (13-17) | Lymphocytes | 8,652 | (1,500-7,000) |
| MCHC g/dl | 33 | (30-36) | Monocytes | 2,472 | (0-850) |
| | | | Eosinophils | ---- | (0-750) |

| | | |
|---|---|---|
| TPP g/dl | 8.1 | (6.0-7.5) |
| Platelets/ul | 410,000 | (>300,000) |
| Reticulocytes% | 0.3 | (<0.6%) |
| Absolute Retic/ul | 19,800 | (<80,000) |
| Plasma color | Normal | |

Toxic neutrophils    1+

**RBC Morphology:** Normal

## Discussion/Interpretation

In light of clinical dehydration, the cat is normoproteinemic and is more anemic than the measured PCV would indicate. The anemia is mild and appears nonregenerative because of the normal reticulocyte count and RBC morphology. There is a marked leukocytosis due to a neutrophilia, pronounced left shift, lymphocytosis and monocytosis. Dohle bodies in neutrophils indicate toxic change. This leukogram is consistent with either chronic granulocytic leukemia or chronic inflammation that involves a major organ or body cavity. The latter was confirmed by abdominal radiographs which revealed pyometra. The decrease in PCV is due to the anemia of inflammation.

The marked leukocyte response in this case was caused by chronic suppuration. This pattern is called a leukemoid reaction since the hematologic features are very similar to chronic granulocytic leukemia. Large internal abscesses, suppurative pyoderma, or suppuration of body cavities are frequent causes.

**Diagnosis** Pyometra with leukemoid reaction and anemia of inflammation.

## NOTES

# CASE 18 Canine 10 Year Old Female Sheltie

**History** Depression, anorexia, pot-bellied abdomen.

**Physical Examination** Normal body temperature, increased pulse, pale mucous membranes, large abdominal mass, marked weight loss.

| | Patient | Reference Range | | Patient | Reference Range |
|---|---|---|---|---|---|
| PCV % | 19 | (37-55) | WBC/ul | 134,000 | (6,000-17,000) |
| Hgb g/dl | 5.6 | (12-15) | Neutrophils | 64,320 | (3,000-11,400) |
| RBC x10⁶/ul | 2.8 | (5.5-8.5) | Band cells | 48,240 | (0-300) |
| MCV fl | 68 | (60-77) | Metamyelocytes | 8,040 | (0) |
| MCH pg | 20 | (19-24) | Myelocytes | 1,340 | (0) |
| MCHC g/dl | 34 | (32-36) | Lymphocytes | 8,040 | (1,000-4,800) |
| | | | Monocytes | 2,680 | (150-1,350) |
| | | | Eosinophils | ---- | (100-750) |
| | | | Blasts | Few | |

| | | |
|---|---|---|
| TPP g/dl | 6.4 | (6.0-7.5) |
| Plasma color | Normal | |
| Reticulocytes % | 0.2 | (<1.0) |
| Absolute Retic/ul | 5,600 | (<80,000) |
| Platelets/uL | 23,000 | (>200,000) |
| NRBC | 3/100WBC | |

**RBC morphology:** Normal

## Discussion/Interpretation

A severe thrombocytopenia and normocytic normochromic anemia are present. A marked neutrophilic leukocytosis is present with a severe left shift that includes metamyelocytes and myelocytes. Toxic change was not evident but blast cells that appeared to be granulocytic precursors were detected (Figures C18-1 and C18-2). Lymphocytes and monocytes are increased. In an intact female dog, the leukocyte pattern could be indicative of chronic inflammation as would occur in a closed pyometra. The severe anemia, thrombocytopenia, and excessive number of immature neutrophils are strong indication for bone marrow aspiration. The abdominal mass was a very large spleen. The bone marrow and spleen aspirates were diffusely infiltrated by large blast cells and developing neutrophil precursors (Figures C18-3 and C18-4). Megakaryocytes and erythroid precursors were rare. Similar cells were detected in aspirates of lymph node. These findings confirmed a diagnosis of chronic granulocytic leukemia.

**Diagnosis** Chronic granulocytic leukemia. The leukocyte pattern is similar to that which is found in dogs with extensive suppurative inflammation. However, in chronic granulocytic leukemia, a disproportionate number of immature neutrophils is often noted along with severe anemia and thrombocytopenia due to myelophthisis.

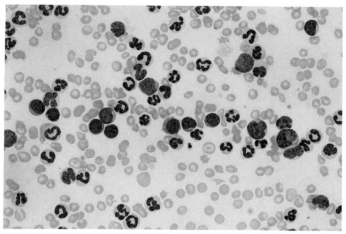

**Figure C18-1**
Canine blood. Marked leukocytosis due to a neutrophilia and a population of large round cells that are difficult to identify at this magnification (40x).

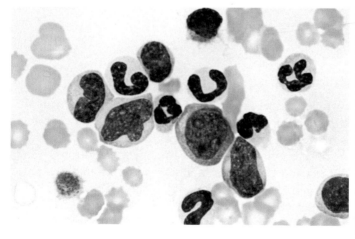

**Figure C18-2**
Canine blood. Segmented neutrophils are present but there is a disproportionate number of immature granulocytes present with indented, lobulated, or rounded nuclei. One of the larger cells is a blast form and has multiple nucleoli. RBCs are normocytic and normochromic indicating a nonregenerative anemia. Platelets are markedly reduced. These findings are consistent with chronic granulocytic leukemia (100x).

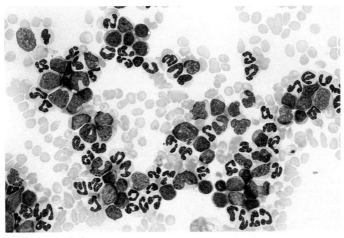

## Figure C18-3
Bone marrow. The marrow is cellular and contains numerous large immature granulocytes and mature neutrophils. Erythroid and megakaryocytic precursors are rare (40x).

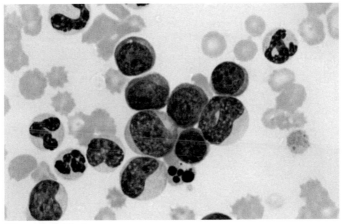

## Figure C18-4
Bone marrow. Higher magnification reveals an abundance of blast cells that have a light blue cytoplasm, round or elongate nucleus, and prominent nucleoli. Toxic change is not apparent in either blood or bone marrow neutrophils (100x).

# NOTES

# CASE 19 Feline 4 Year Old Male DSH

**History** Loss of appetite and lethargy for 3 days.

**Physical Examination** T=104°F, pale mucous membranes, mild dehydration.

|  | Patient | Reference Range |  | Patient | Reference Range |
|---|---|---|---|---|---|
| PCV % | 19 | (30-40) | WBC/ul | 7,100 | (5,500-19,500) |
| Hgb g/dl | 5.8 | (8.5-15) | Neutrophils | 3,479 | (2,500-12,500) |
| RBC x10⁶/ul | 2.9 | (5.2-10) | Band cells | 71 | (0-300) |
| MCV fl | 67 | (39-55) | Lymphocytes | 3,124 | (1,500-7,000) |
| MCH pg | 14 | (13-17) | Monocytes | 426 | (0-850) |
| MCHC g/dl | 31 | (30-36) | Eosinophils | ---- | (0-750) |
| TPP g/dl | 7.9 | (6.0-7.5) |  |  |  |
| Platelets/ul | ADQ | (>300,000) |  |  |  |
| Reticulocytes % | 9.0 | (<0.6%) |  |  |  |
| Absolute Retic/ul | 279,900 | (<80,000) |  |  |  |
| Plasma color | Icteric |  |  |  |  |
| NRBC | 46/100WBC |  |  |  |  |

**RBC Morphology**
Anisocytosis 3+
Macrocytosis 2+
Polychromasia 3+
Howell Jolly Bodies 2+
Agglutination 2+
Numerous *Haemobartonella felis*

## Discussion/Interpretation

A severe regenerative anemia is present with a slightly increased TPP. The regenerative response is orderly and proportional to the severity of anemia and is characterized by anisocytosis, macrocytosis, increased MCV, polychromasia, reticulocytosis, and metarubricytosis (Figure C19-1). The absence of hypoproteinemia and clinical hemorrhage, and the presence of an intense regenerative response, icteric plasma, and agglutination are consistent with hemolytic anemia. Causes of hemolytic anemia include infectious agents, immune-mediated disease, toxins, fragmentation, and osmotic lysis. The identification of numerous *H. felis* organisms on erythrocytes (Figure C19-2) coupled with the regenerative response confirms a diagnosis of Haemobartonellosis. These parasites initiate immune-mediated destruction of RBCs which frequently results in a positive direct Coombs' test.

The number of organisms on the smear can change dramatically from day to day. Thus, if the parasite is suspected, repeated examinations of blood films may be necessary to make a diagnosis. Organisms may detach from erythrocytes if there is a time delay between blood collection and preparation of the blood film. Detached organisms may aggregate at the feather edge of the smear.

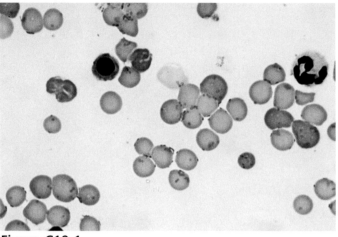

**Figure C19-1**
Feline blood. Marked polychromasia, anisocytosis, and macrocytosis indicate regenerative anemia. Small basophilic coccoid or rod-shaped organisms are noted on the RBCs. A few ring forms with a light central area can be seen on a few RBCs. These organisms are *Haemobartonella felis* which causes a hemolytic anemia (100x).

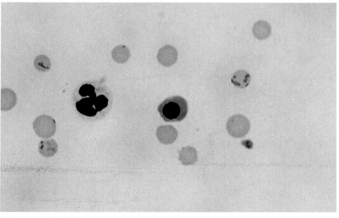

**Figure C19-2**
Feline blood. In a thin area of the smear, the ring forms of the parasite are visible in small chains or groups on the RBC membrane (100x).

# CASE 20  Canine 9 Year Old Female Golden Retriever

**History**  Weakness, lethargy, weight loss for 5 weeks.

**Physical Examination**  Dog is alert but very weak; pale mucous membranes, enlarged liver and spleen, systolic heart murmur.

|  | Patient | Reference Range |  | Patient | Reference Range |
|---|---|---|---|---|---|
| PCV % | 11 | (37-55) | WBC/ul | 5,800 | (6,000-17,000) |
| Hgb g/dl | 3.8 | (12-15) | Neutrophils | 812 | (3,000-11,400) |
| RBC x10⁶/ul | 1.7 | (5.5-8.5) | Band cells | ---- | (0-300) |
| MCV fl | 64 | (60-77) | Lymphocytes | 3,248 | 1,000-4,800) |
| MCH pg | 24 | (19-24) | Monocytes | 232 | (150-1,350) |
| MCHC g/dl | 35 | (32-36) | Eosinophils | ---- | (100-750) |
|  |  |  | Blasts | 1,508 |  |

| | | |
|---|---|---|
| TPP g/dl | 7.2 | (6.0-7.5) |
| Plasma color | Normal | |
| Reticulocytes % | 0.5 | (<1.0) |
| Absolute Retic/ul | 8,500 | (<80,000) |
| Platelets/uL | 19,000 | (>200,000) |

**RBC morphology**
No abnormalities

### Discussion/Interpretation

The anemia is normocytic and normochromic with an absence of reticulocytosis or polychromasia (Figure C20-1). These features indicate that the anemia is nonregenerative. The combination of severe nonregenerative anemia, thrombocytopenia, and neutropenia is called pancytopenia. The neutropenia is not accompanied by a left shift. Causes of this hematologic pattern include infectious agents, marrow injury due to toxins or drugs, immune-mediated disease, and neoplasia. Bone marrow aspiration is indicated because of the pancytopenia and the blast cells identified in the differential count (Figures C20-1 and C20-2). The marrow aspirate was very cellular and contained a homogenous population of blast cells similar to those in blood (Figure C20-3). These cells were very large and had dark blue cytoplasm, round or indented nuclei, and singular prominent nucleoli. Erythroid, megakaryocytic, or granulocytic precursors were rare.

**Diagnosis**  Acute leukemia. Spleen and liver were diffusely infiltrated with blast cells.

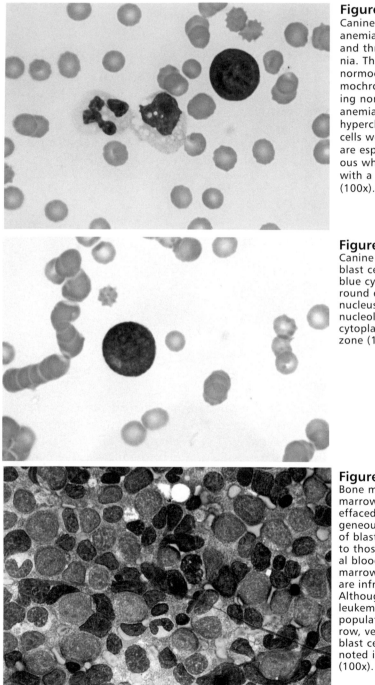

**Figure C20-1**
Canine blood. Severe anemia, leukopenia and thrombocytopenia. The RBC are normocytic and normochromic indicating nonregenerative anemia.Several large hyperchromatic blast cells were noted and are especially obvious when compared with a neutrophil (100x).

**Figure C20-2**
Canine blood. Large blast cell has dark blue cytoplasm, round eccentric nucleus, multiple nucleoli, and focal cytoplasmic clear zone (100x).

**Figure C20-3**
Bone marrow. The marrow has been effaced by a homogeneous population of blast cells similar to those in peripheral blood. Normal marrow precursors are infrequent. Although this acute leukemia has overpopulated the marrow, very few of the blast cells were noted in the CBC (100x).

# NOTES

# NOTES

# CASE 21 Canine 2 Year Old Standard Poodle

**History** Seems to be short of breath and listless. No clinical evidence of dehydration.

**Physical Examination** Normal temperature, rapid pulse (110/minute), mucous membranes are brick red, congested, and sometimes cyanotic. Retinal, scleral, sublingual, and jugular veins are very large and engorged.

| | Patient | Reference Range | | Patient | Reference Range |
|---|---|---|---|---|---|
| PCV % | 78 | (37-55) | WBC/ul | 10,300 | (6,000-17,000) |
| Hgb g/dl | 25.7 | (12-15) | Neutrophils | 6,180 | (3,000-11,400) |
| RBC x10⁶/ul | 12.0 | (5.5-8.5) | Band cells | ---- | (0-300) |
| MCV fl | 65 | (60-77) | Lymphocytes | 2,781 | 1,000-4,800) |
| MCH pg | 20 | (19-24) | Monocytes | 721 | (150-1,350) |
| MCHC g/dl | 33 | (32-36) | Eosinophils | 618 | (100-750) |
| TPP g/dl | 7.5 | (6.0-7.5) | | | |
| Plasma color | Normal | | | | |
| Reticulocytes % | ---- | (<1.0) | | | |
| Platelets/uL | 180,000 | (>200,000) | | | |
| NRBC | 2/100WBC | | | | |

**RBC Morphology**
Anisocytosis 1+
Polychromasia 1+

## Discussion/Interpretation

A PCV of 78% in the absence of severe dehydration indicates an absolute polycythemia. Absolute polycythemias are classified as primary or secondary according to the cause or mechanism. Primary polycythemia is a myeloproliferative disorder or neoplasm characterized by excessive production of mature RBCs, normal arterial oxygen content, and normal or decreased erythropoietin levels. Secondary polycythemias are caused by hypoxemia which leads to increased erythropoietin levels. Secondary polycythemias can also be caused by excess production of erythropoietin in the absence of hypoxemia. The latter is quite rare and occurs with tumors, cysts, or space-occupying lesions of the kidney, liver, or adrenal. Chest radiographs of the Poodle revealed a pumpkin-shaped cardiac silhouette. Severe hypoxemia was confirmed by the arterial blood gas analysis ($PO_2$ = 32 mmHg, reference range 85-95 mmHg). Angiography revealed a large interventricular septal defect that allowed right to left shunting of blood. Hypoxemia resulted because a large portion of systemic venous blood bypassed the lungs. The reduced arterial oxygen content was detected by receptors in the kidney that initiated an increase in erythropoietin. This hormone is the primary stimulus for marrow erythroid hyperplasia (Figure C21-1).

**Diagnosis** Absolute polycythemia secondary to hypoxemia due to cardiac defect.

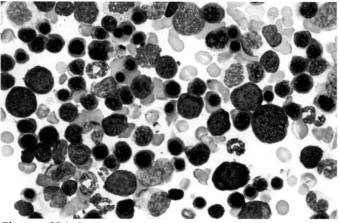

**Figure C21-1**
Bone marrow. The severe polycythemia in this dog is caused by overproduction of RBCs in the marrow. This is confirmed by the marked erythroid hyperplasia that is evident. The maturation is orderly and there is no evidence of neoplasia. Chronic hypoxemia caused increased erythropoietin secretion which resulted in polycythemia (40x).

## CASE 22 Canine 6 Year Old Male English Bull Dog

**History** Prior history of otitis which responded to treatment. Mild anemia and increase in TPP noted at that time. Presented 3 months later with enlarged peripheral lymph nodes and decreased activity level.

**Physical Examination** Weight loss and enlargement of all palpable lymph nodes; normal body temperature; no evidence of dehydration.

| | Patient | Reference Range | | Patient | Reference Range |
|---|---|---|---|---|---|
| PCV % | 30 | (37-55) | WBC/ul | 13,800 | (6,000-17,000) |
| Hgb g/dl | 10.2 | (12-15) | Neutrophils | 11,454 | (3,000-11,400) |
| RBC x10⁶/ul | 4.5 | (5.5-8.5) | Band cells | ---- | (0-300) |
| MCV fl | 67 | (60-77) | Lymphocytes | 690 | 1,000-4,800) |
| MCH pg | 20 | (19-24) | Monocytes | 1,380 | (150-1,350) |
| MCHC g/dl | 34 | (32-36) | Eosinophils | 138 | (100-750) |
| TPP g/dl | 10 | (6.0-7.5) | | | |
| Plasma color | Normal | | | | |
| Reticulocytes % | 0.5 | (<1.0) | | | |
| Absolute Retic/ul | 22,500 | (<80,000) | | | |
| Platelets/uL | ADQ | (>200,000) | | | |

**RBC morphology**
No abnormalities

### Discussion/Interpretation

A mild normocytic, normochromic anemia is present with no evidence of regeneration. PCVs in Bull Dogs fall in the upper end of the reference range because they are a brachycephalic breed. The absence of dehydration suggests that the hyperproteinemia is due to hyperglobulinemia. The PCV and TPP values are similar to previous measurements indicating that these changes are persistent. The leukogram suggests a stress response or mild inflammation. Atypical lymphocytes were not detected on the blood films. Basophilic background on the blood film is consistent with hyperproteinemia (Figure C22-1). Fine needle aspiration of lymph nodes and protein electrophoresis are indicated.

Causes of generalized lymph node enlargement include lymphoma, systemic infection, and immune-mediated disease. The lymph node aspirate revealed a homogenous population of large lymphoblasts and confirmed a diagnosis of lymphoma. Bone marrow aspiration revealed a similar infiltrate (Figure C22-2). A monoclonal gammopathy was evident in the serum protein electrophoresis and was responsible for the hyperproteinemia. Lymphoid neoplasms may produce very high levels of a single immunoglobulin which causes a monoclonal peak in the electrophoresis. Most dogs with lymphoma do not have significant hematologic abnormalities. The most frequent changes are mild nonregenerative anemia and a mature neutrophilia. Both changes are due to the presence of a neoplasm. An absolute lymphocytosis in canine or feline lymphoma is an infrequent occurrence.

**Diagnosis**  Lymphoma with monoclonal gammopathy.

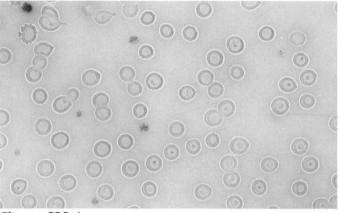

**Figure C22-1**
Canine Blood. Marked hyperproteinemia produces a heavy blue background that highlights the cell membranes of the RBCs. RBC morphology does not reveal any evidence of regeneration. Platelets are reduced (100x).

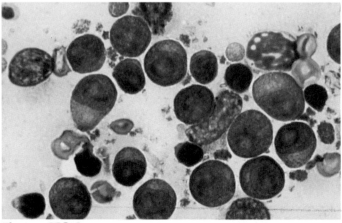

**Figure C22-2**
Bone marrow. Normal granulopoietic and erythroid cells have been replaced by a population of large lymphoblasts that have singular prominent nucleoli (100x).

## CASE 23 Canine 9 Year Old Castrated Male Mixed Breed

**History** Treated for anemia with hematinics for 2 weeks. Moderate weight loss. Anorexia and profound weakness for 2 days. Distended abdomen.

**Physical Examination** Normal body temperature; pale mucous membranes and rapid respiration. Abdominocentesis reveals a large amount of bloody fluid. Dog is very weak and collapsed.

| | Patient | Reference Range | | Patient | Reference Range |
|---|---|---|---|---|---|
| PCV % | 22 | (37-55) | WBC/ul | 28,100 | (6,000-17,000) |
| Hgb g/dl | 6.8 | (12-18) | Neutrophils | 23,323 | (3,000-11,400) |
| RBC x10⁶/ul | 2.68 | (5.5-8.5) | Band cells | 562 | (0-300) |
| MCV fl | 79 | (60-77) | Lymphocytes | 1,124 | 1,000-4,800) |
| MCH pg | 25 | (19-24) | Monocytes | 3,091 | (150-1,350) |
| MCHC g/dl | 31 | (32-36) | Eosinophils | ---- | (100-750) |
| | | | | | |
| TPP g/dl | 5.1 | (6.0-7.5) | | | |
| Plasma color | Normal | | | | |
| Reticulocytes % | 19 | (<1.0) | | | |
| Absolute Retic/ul | 509,000 | (<80,000) | | | |
| Platelets/uL | 99,000 | (>200,000) | | | |
| NRBC | 28/100WBC | | | | |

**RBC morphology**
    Anisocytosis, Polychromasia, Poilkilocytosis 3+
    Macrocytosis, Acanthocytosis 2+
    Schistocytes, Howell Jolly bodies 1+

### Discussion/Interpretation

A marked regenerative anemia is present as evidenced by anisocytosis, polychromasia, reticulocytosis, metarubricytosis, and an increase in MCV and a decrease in MCHC. Hypoproteinemia, the absence of icterus, and the abdominal hemorrhage confirm blood loss anemia of several days duration. A coagulation profile revealed a moderate increase in prothrombin time, partial thromboplastin time, and fibrin degradation products. These changes along with moderate thrombocytopenia and schistocytes (Figure C23-3) indicate the presence of disseminated intravascular coagulation. The leukogram reveals a moderate neutrophilia, mild left shift, and monocytosis that are consistent with inflammation and tissue necrosis. Acanthocytes are numerous on the blood film (Figure C23-1 and C23-2) and are frequently associated with hemangiosarcoma in the liver. The CBC results, history, and abdominal hemorrhage are compatible with hemangiosarcoma.

**Diagnosis** Hemorrhagic anemia and DIC with inflammatory leukogram. Exploratory surgery was done. A ruptured splenic hemangiosarcoma with numerous metastatic lesions in the liver was detected.

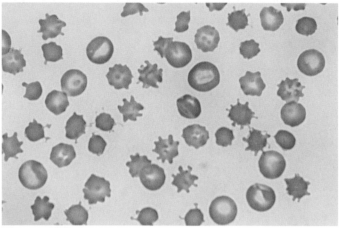

**Figure C23-1**
Canine blood. Anisocytosis, polychromasia, and macrocytosis indicate regenerative anemia. Marked poikilocytosis is due to the presence of numerous acanthocytes. These RBCs have irregular membrane projections that have variable lengths and rounded points. Platelet numbers are reduced (100x).

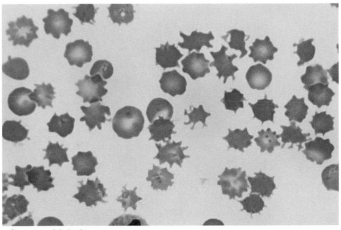

**Figure C23-2**
Canine blood. Numerous acanthocytes and spheroechinocytes are present. Acanthocytes in a dog with anemia and thrombocytopenia suggest that hepatic involvement with hemangiosarcoma should be considered (100x).

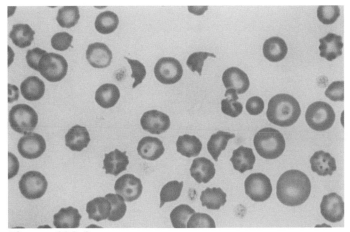

**Figure C23-3**
Canine blood. Marked thrombocytopenia and the presence of several schistocytes or fragmented RBCs are indications that thrombosis or DIC is occurring. Coagulation tests are indicated (100x).

# NOTES

# CASE 24 Canine 9 Year Old Spayed Female Corgi

**History** Bloody urine and weakness for 5 days.

**Physical Examination** Mucous membranes are pale and melena is present. Numerous petechial hemorrhages. Abdomen is painful on palpation.

| | Patient | Reference Range | | Patient | Reference Range |
|---|---|---|---|---|---|
| PCV % | 24 | (37-55) | WBC/ul | 44,900 | (6,000-17,000) |
| Hgb g/dl | 8.4 | (12-18) | Neutrophils | 34.124 | (3,000-11,400) |
| RBC x10⁶/ul | 2.67 | (5.5-8.5) | Band cells | 4,939 | (0-300) |
| MCV fl | 90 | (60-77) | Lymphocytes | 898 | (1,000-4,800) |
| MCH pg | 31.5 | (19-24) | Monocytes | 3,143 | (150-1,350) |
| MCHC g/dl | 34 | (32-36) | Eosinophils | 1,347 | (100-750) |
| TPP g/dl | 5.0 | (6.0-7.5) | | | |
| Plasma color | Normal | | | | |
| Reticulocytes % | 8 | (<1.0) | | | |
| Absolute Retic/ul | 480,600 | (<80,000) | | | |
| Platelets/uL | 3,000 | (>200,000) | | | |
| NRBC | | 34/100WBC | | | |

**RBC Morphology**
Anisocytosis, polychromasia, macrocytosis 3+

**Discussion/Interpretation**

Macrocytosis, reticulocytosis, polychromasia, metarubricytosis, and anisocytosis indicate regenerative anemia. Hypoproteinemia, hematuria, petechiation, and melena indicate that the anemia is due to hemorrhage as a result of the severe thrombocytopenia (Figure C24-1). Hemolytic anemia is also a possibility. A neutrophilic leukocytosis with left shift and monocytosis indicate inflammation with possible tissue necrosis. Lymphopenia is due to stress. The eosinophilia if persistent is an indication of hypersensitivity. A coagulation profile (PT, PTT, FDP) was normal. Direct Coombs' test and titers for Ehrlichia, Lyme disease, and Rocky Mountain Spotted Fever were negative.

Aspiration of bone marrow is indicated to assess thrombopoiesis. The marrow was very cellular and revealed an increase in immature and mature megakaryocytes (Figure C24-2). Erythroid hyperplasia was also noted. These findings indicate that the thrombocytopenia was due to excessive destruction rather than reduced production.

**Diagnosis** Presumptive immune-mediated thrombocytopenia. Dog was treated successfully with predisone and azothioprine.

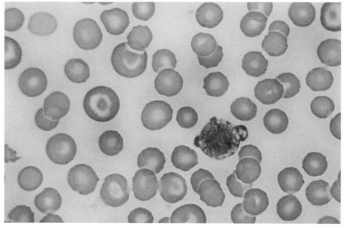

**Figure C24-1**
Canine blood. Regenerative anemia and thrombocytopenia are pronounced. The large round granular structure in the center is a giant platelet. Large shreds of megakaryocyte cytoplasm are often found in severely thrombocytopenic animals (100x).

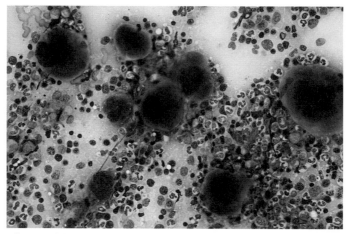

**Figure C24-2**
Bone marrow. Bone marrow examination is helpful in the assessment of thrombocytopenic animals. In this marrow there are numerous megakaryocytes in the field indicating that the decrease in platelets is due to accelerated destruction rather than decreased production (25x).

# NOTES

# NOTES

# CASE 25 Canine 11 Year Old Spayed Female Basset Hound

**History** Dog presented for suture removal and recheck following a splenectomy that was done 8 days ago. Hemoperitoneum and a large splenic hematoma were noted during laparotomy. PCV at the time of surgery was 25%.

**Physical Examination** Abdominal incision is healing normally. TPR is normal. Mucous membranes are pink with normal capillary refill.

| | Patient | Reference Range | | Patient | Reference Range |
|---|---|---|---|---|---|
| PCV % | 30 | (37-55) | WBC/ul | 7,000 | (6,000-17,000) |
| Hgb g/dl | 10.7 | (12-18) | Neutrophils | 5,600 | (3,000-11,400) |
| RBC x10⁶/ul | 4.9 | (5.5-8.5) | Band cells | ---- | (0-300) |
| MCV fl | 62 | (60-77) | Lymphocytes | 630 | (1,000-4,800) |
| MCH pg | 22 | (19-24) | Monocytes | 560 | (150-1,350) |
| MCHC g/dl | 35 | (32-36) | Eosinophils | 140 | (100-750) |
| TPP g/dl | 7.0 | (6.0-7.5) | | | |
| Plasma color | Normal | | | | |
| Reticulocytes % | 1.3 | (<1.0) | | | |
| Absolute Retic/ul | 63,700 | (<80,000) | | | |
| Platelets/uL | ADQ | (>200,000) | | | |

**RBC morphology**
Polychromasia 1+

## Discussion/Interpretation

The leukogram is unremarkable except for a lymphopenia that is due to stress. A mild, normocytic, normochromic anemia is present with a minimal reticulocyte response. These findings indicate that the regenerative response is either inadequate or subsiding as the PCV approaches normalcy. Examination of the blood film is indicated in all anemic animals. Erythrocytes need to be examined for size, shape, color, and inclusions. Examination of the blood film revealed moderate numbers of coccoid, basophilic, epicellular RBC parasites (Figure C25-1). Many of the organisms were arranged in chains that branched. The morphology of the organisms was consistent with *Haemobartonella canis*.

*H. canis* causes mild anemia due to extravascular hemolysis in dogs that have been splenectomized or in those that have received glucocorticoids, chemotherapy, or immunosuppressive drugs. The organism can be transmitted by blood transfusion or by biting arthropods. This dog received a blood transfusion during surgery and the donor was subsequently identified as an infected carrier.

**Diagnosis**  Mild anemia due to *Haemobartonella canis*. Dog was treated with tetracycline and made an uneventful recovery.

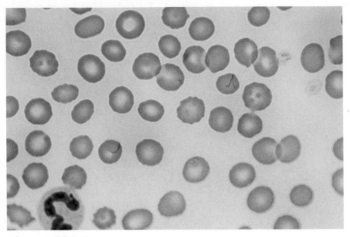

**Figure C25-1**
Canine blood. Chains of basophilic small coccoid organisms are noted on the surface of two RBCs. *Haemobartonella canis* causes a mild to moderate hemolytic anemia in dogs that have been splenectomized or treated with immunosuppressive drugs.

# CASE 26   Feline 7 Year Old Male Domestic Shorthair

**History**   Owner reports that the cat drinks a lot of water and has been losing weight. Appetite is diminished.

**Physical Examination**   Cat is depressed, mildly dehydrated, and in poor body condition.

| | Patient | Reference Range | | Patient | Reference Range |
|---|---|---|---|---|---|
| PCV % | 20 | (30-40) | WBC/ul | 8,000 | (5,500-19,500) |
| Hgb g/dl | 6.8 | (8.5-15) | Neutrophils | 7,200 | (2,500-12,500) |
| RBC x10⁶/ul | 4.0 | (5.2-10) | Band cells | ---- | (0-300) |
| MCV fl | 50 | (39-55) | Lymphocytes | 560 | (1,500-7,000) |
| MCH pg | 17 | (13-17) | Monocytes | 240 | (0-850) |
| MCHC g/dl | 34 | (30-36) | Eosinophils | ---- | (0-750) |
| TPP g/dl | 7.9 | (6.0-7.5) | | | |
| Platelets/ul | ADQ | (>300,000) | | | |
| Reticulocytes % | 0.4 | (<0.6%) | | | |
| Absolute Retic/ul | 16,000 | (80,000) | | | |
| Plasma color | Normal | | | | |

**RBC Morphology**
   Few Heinz bodies

**Discussion/Interpretation**

The CBC reveals a moderate, normocytic, normochromic anemia with no evidence of regeneration. Hyperproteinemia is due to dehydration. The leukogram reveals a marked lymphopenia which can be due to stress or to loss or sequestration of lymphocytes. Examples of the latter include chylous effusions or protein-losing enteropathy. Absence of GI signs and negative chest radiograph eliminates these causes. Examination of the blood film did not reveal significant abnormalities.

A bone marrow aspirate revealed a cellular marrow with an increased M:E ratio, normal iron stores, and adequate megakaryocytes. Maturation in granulocytes and in the limited number of erythroid cells was normal. In light of the normal neutrophil count and the moderate non-regenerative anemia, the M:E ratio is increased due to decreased erythroid activity rather than increased granulopoiesis (Figure 26-1). Causes of erythroid depression need to be considered. Serum chemistry results indicate severe azotemia (urea=205 mg/dl, creatinine=11.9 mg/dl). Isosthenuria and severe proteinuria with an inactive sediment were noted in the urinalysis. The azotemia and urine specific gravity were unaffected by fluid therapy and diuresis. These findings are consistent with chronic renal disease with severe proteinuria. The anemia is due to diminished erythropoietin production which causes decreased RBC production in the bone marrow. In the absence of a regenerative anemia or certain metabolic disorders, Heinz bodies are considered an incidental finding.

**Diagnosis** Nonregenerative anemia due to chronic renal disease (renal amyloidosis)

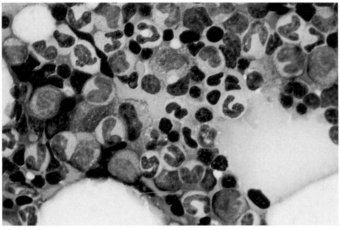

### Figure C26-1
Feline bone marrow. In nonregenerative anemias, bone marrow assessment is extremely valuable in deciding the cause or mechanism. In this cat, diminished erythropoietin levels as a result of renal disease lead to erythroid hypoplasia. Therefore the M:E ratio is increased in the marrow due to a reduction in erythroid cells relative to the granulocytes (40x).

# CASE 27 Canine 12 Year Old Mixed Breed Male

**History** Male dog was admitted to the hospital 4 days ago for elective castration due to benign prostatic hypertrophy. There was no palpable tumor but the prostate was symmetrically enlarged and the dog was having difficulty urinating and defecating. He had previously been in excellent health and had an unremarkable medical history. He had no past history of bleeding. Surgery had been uneventful but petechiae and ecchymoses on the ventral abdomen were noted four days postoperatively.

| | Patient | Reference Range | | Patient | Reference Range |
|---|---|---|---|---|---|
| PCV % | 44 | (37-55) | WBC (corrected) /ul | 2,200 | (6,000-17,500) |
| Hb g/dl | 14 | (12-18) | Neutrophils | 800 | (3,000-11,500) |
| RBC x10⁶/ul | 6.2 | (6-8) | Band cells | 0 | (0-400) |
| MCV fl | 71 | (60-77) | Lymphocytes | 1,200 | (1,000-4,800) |
| MCHC g/dl | 34 | (31-35) | Monocytes | 200 | (150-1,350) |
| MCH pg | 22.5 | (19-24) | Eosinophils | 0 | (100-1,250) |
| | | | Basophils | 0 | (0) |

| | Patient | Reference Range |
|---|---|---|
| TPP g/dl | 7.3 | (6.0-8.0) |
| Platelets/ul | 35,000 | (200-400) |
| Platelet morphology | Some oval, large | |

| Coagulation Tests | Patient | Reference Range |
|---|---|---|
| Thrombin time (TT) sec | 12 | (12 - control) |
| PT sec | 11 | (12 - control) |
| APTT sec | 18 | (18 - control) |

PT is Prothrombin Time; APTT is Activated Partial Thromboplastin Time. With coagulation tests, patient values differing by more than 30% of the control value are considered significant.

## Discussion/Interpretation

The hemogram reveals severe thrombocytopenia and leukopenia. The leukopenia is characterized by neutropenia. Because a left shift is not present, the neutropenia is most likely due to a problem in marrow production. Tests of secondary hemostasis, coagulation appear appropriate.

Causes of concurrent neutropenia and thrombocytopenia should be considered. In light of the patient's recent history and the acuteness of this presentation, drug and infectious etiologies should be considered. While awaiting the results of rickettsial serologic tests, appropriate antimicrobial therapy should be initiated, especially considering this patient's significant neutropenia. Bone marrow examination should be considered.

This patient was no longer receiving drugs at the time of this presentation. *Ehrlichia* titers were markedly elevated. The patient responded well to appropriate therapy. This is an example of immune-mediated thrombocytopenia secondary to an infectious process.

# CASE 28 Canine 7 Year Old Mixed Breed Spayed Female

**History** An urgent consultation was requested for a patient in the intensive care unit. This dog had returned from surgery following extensive bowel resection for sarcoma. During surgery she was autotransfused from vacuumed abdominal blood. Over the 24 hour postoperative period she had received three units of crossmatch compatible whole blood (of the same blood type as hers) for extensive intraoperative and postoperative blood loss. Following surgery, continued bleeding followed by oozing was observed from the abdominal drain tube and following venipuncture. There was no previous history of bleeding and a hemostatic profile performed 24 hours presurgically was similar to control values. Petechiae and purpura were noted on the lower limbs. Chest radiographs were normal and blood culture was negative.

| | Patient | Reference Range | | Patient | Reference Range |
|---|---|---|---|---|---|
| PCV % | 22 | (37-55) | WBC (corrected)/ul | 10800 | (6,000-17,500) |
| Hb g/dl | 7.6 | (12-18) | Neutrophils | 7750 | (3,000-11,500) |
| RBC x10⁶/ul | 3.2 | (6-8) | Band cells | 750 | (0-400) |
| MCV fl | 65 | (60-77) | Lymphocytes | 1300 | (1,000-4,800) |
| MCHC g/dl | 31.5 | (31-35) | Monocytes | 900 | (150-1,350) |
| MCH pg | 20 | (19-24) | Eosinophils | 100 | (100-1,250) |
| Reticulocytes % | 0 | (0-1.5) | Basophils | 0 | (0) |
| TPP g/dl | 5.7 | (6.0-8.0) | | | |
| Fibrinogen mg/dl | 200 | (200-400) | | | |
| Platelets/ul | 23,000 | (200,000-400,000) | | | |
| NRBC | 4/100WBC | | | | |

**Morphology**
RBC Poik/leptocytes
WBC Toxic neutrophils
Platelet Many large

**Coagulation Tests**
| | | |
|---|---|---|
| Thrombin time (TT) sec | 20 | (12-control) |
| PT sec | 19 | (12-control) |
| APTT sec | 31 | (18-control) |
| FDP ug/ml | 0 | (<10) |
| Antithrombin III % | 71 | (>85) |
| D-dimers | 10 | (0) |

D-dimers are specific fibrin(ogen) degradation products using a canine specific test.

**Discussion/Interpretation**

This patient appears to have an acute blood loss anemia which is severe, normocytic, normochromic and nonresponsive. The presence of nucleated red cells, in this case metarubricytes, may be considered an acute response. There is a marked reduction in plasma proteins when considering both the reference interval and the patient's age. (Older dogs have higher total protein concentrations than younger dogs.) The platelet count is markedly reduced. The presence of large platelets may be an acute and positive response to the patient's thrombocytopenia.

This patient is in DIC. DIC is always secondary to a significant primary process. The possibilities of inducing DIC in this patient include the surgical trauma, the presence of neoplasia, and the possibility, despite all efforts, of a transfusion reaction.

# CASE 29 Canine 5 Year Old Mixed Breed Intact Male

**History** At 2100 hours this patient was bitten on his left forepaw, around the toes, by Crotalus atrox, the Western Diamond Back rattlesnake. He was brought to an emergency clinic within 40 minutes. There he was noted to have pain and swelling limited to the left front leg, mostly the paw region. Vital signs were normal. The leg was immobilized and an intravenous line was started in the right foreleg. During the evening the swelling was noted to extend up the left leg and pain extended to the left axillary area. The next day he developed abdominal pain and one episode of emesis occurred. On that morning, after skin testing, ten vials of antivenin (*Crotalidae*) polyvalent were administered over several hours. The following day the dog was discharged with oral pain medication. He regained full use of his paw and leg. The table contains the notable laboratory results.

| | | Patient | | | Reference Range |
|---|---|---|---|---|---|
| Test | Day 1 | | Day 2 | Day 3 | |
| Time | 2200 | 0400 | 2200 | 1000 | |
| Hb g/dl | 14.0 | 12.9 | 12.2 | 11.5 | (12-18) |
| PCV % | 40.0 | 37.7 | 35.3 | 28.8 | (37-55) |
| Platelets/ul | ND | 30000 | 115000 | 196000 | (200-400) |
| PT sec | 11.5 | >120 | 13.0 | 11.9 | (12-control) |
| APTT sec | 35.9 | >120 | 30.4 | 28.8 | (18-control) |
| Fibrinogen mg/dl | 100 | <50 | <50 | 240 | (200-400) |

## Discussion/Interpretation

This patient's progressive modest anemia reflects fluid therapy. At initial presentation the patient did have a low fibrinogen concentration. Six hours later fibrinogen was not detectable, platelet count was markedly reduced and PT and APTT were prolonged. Within 24 hours of presentation the patient exhibited clinical improvement which was corroborated by the laboratory tests.

This is a case of DIC secondary to snake envenomation. It is interesting to follow these tests over time, especially with success.

# NOTES

# 13
# Self-Test Questions

# QUESTIONS

1. Which of the following is incorrect ?
   A. Erythropoietin stimulates red blood cell (RBC) production
   B. Erythropoietin stimulates white blood cell (WBC) production
   C. Erythropoietin stimulates platelet production
   D. Erythropoietin is produced by the kidney
   E. None of the above

2. Which of the following is/are correct?
   A. In normal dogs, erythrocytes circulate for approximately 100 days.
   B. In normal cats, erythrocytes circulate for approximately 80-90 days.
   C. Approximately 1% of the circulating red cells of the dog are replaced daily.
   D. Effete red cells are phagocytized and metabolized by the macrophages of spleen, bone marrow and liver.
   E. All of the above

3. Which of the following is incorrect?
   A. The primary function of the red cell is to carry oxygen to tissue cells and to carry carbon dioxide away.
   B. The primary red cell metabolic pathway is anaerobic glycolysis.
   C. Oxidation of hemoglobin leads to methemoglobinemia and/or Heinz body formation.
   D. Feline hemoglobin is less susceptible to oxidation than canine hemoglobin.
   E. Heinz body formation and Heinz body hemolytic anemia occurs more readily in cats than dogs.

4. The proper term for poikilocytes with 2-10 blunt elongate finger-like surface projections is:
   A. Acanthocytes
   B. Elliptocytes
   C. Eccentrocytes
   D. Schistocytes
   E. Burr cells

5. Which of the following is/are correct ?
   A. Crenation is the least common artifactual change seen in blood films.
   B. Crenation is most often confused with spherocytosis.
   C. Crenation is more prominent in films made from EDTA-anticoagulated blood than in films made from fresh non-anticoagulated blood.
   D. Crenation affects only selected red cells on the blood film where as true poikilocytosis affects all red cells on the blood film.
   E. All of the above.

6. Regenerative anemias:
   A. Are characterized by increased polychromatophils on routinely stained blood films.
   B. Are anemias with reticulocyte counts of greater than 80,000/μl
   C. Are either the result of blood loss or hemolysis.
   D. Are best confirmed by absolute reticulocyte counts
   E. All of the above are correct.

7. Which type of anemia best fits a reticulocyte count of 100,000 reticulocytes/ul and a decreased total plasma protein?
   A. Blood loss anemias
   B. Hemolytic anemias
   C. Cytoplasmic maturation defect anemias
   D. Nuclear maturation defect anemias
   E. Hypoproliferative anemias

8. Conditions which can cause immune-mediated hemolytic disease include:
   A. Heartworm disease
   B. Lymphoma
   C. Lupus erythematosus
   D. Exposure to certain drugs
   E. All of the above

9. Which of the following is correct?
   A. Maturation defect anemias have nonregenerative peripheral blood patterns and erythroid hyperplasia in the bone marrow.
   B. Maturation defect anemias have regenerative peripheral blood patterns and erythroid hyperplasia in the bone marrow.
   C. Maturation defect anemias have nonregenerative peripheral blood patterns and erythroid hypoplasia in the bone marrow.
   D. Maturation defect anemias have regenerative and nonregenerative peripheral blood patterns and myelofibrotic bone marrow.
   E. None of the above.

10. Which of the following is/are incorrect about polycythemia?
    A. Polycythemia is defined as increased circulating red cell mass.
    B. At PCV values >65%, hyperviscosity and poor perfusion and oxygenation of tissues are present.
    C. Transient polycythemia may be caused by splenic contraction.
    D. Polycythemias can be classified as relative, transient, or absolute.
    E. Is most commonly caused by polycythemia vera.

11. Laboratory features of relative polycythemia may include:
    A. Moderate increases in PCV
    B. Elevated total protein concentration
    C. Hypernatremia and hyperchloremia
    D. Concentrated urine specific gravity
    E. All of the above

12. Which of the following is/are correct?
    A. Neutrophils serve as the primary defense against invasion of tissues by microorganisms.
    B. Neutrophils kill bacteria and can also damage or participate in the destruction of mycotic agents, algae, and viruses.
    C. Neutrophils accumulate at sites of inflammation or bacterial infection by a process of directional migration or chemotaxis.
    D. At the site of inflammation, neutrophils are capable of phagocytosis and microbicidal activity.
    E. All of the above

13. Which of the following can affect the neutrophil count in peripheral blood?
    A. Changes in the rates of marrow production and release
    B. Exchange between marginal neutrophil pool and circulating neutrophil pool
    C. Tissue demand
    D. Corticosteroids
    E. All of the above

14. Mechanisms of neutropenia include:
    A. Increased demand or consumption in tissues
    B. Decreased marrow production
    C. Dysgranulopoiesis
    D. Increased movement from the circulating neutrophil pool to the marginal neutrophil pool
    E. All of the above

15. Causes of neutrophilia include all of the following except:
    A. Epinephrine release
    B. Glucorticoid release
    C. Inflammation
    D. Hemorrhage
    E. Endotoxemia

16. Which of the following best describes a leukogram characterized by a mild leukocytosis with mature neutrophilia, lymphopenia, eosinopenia, and mild monocytosis?
    A. Stress leukogram
    B. Acute inflammatory leukogram
    C. Chronic inflammatory leukogram
    D. Leukemoid reaction
    E. Leukemia

17. Which of the following is incorrect about eosinophils?
    A. Eosinophils are produced in the bone marrow in a process similar to neutrophil production.
    B. Eosinophils participate as a major component of systemic hypersensitivity reactions.
    C. Eosinophils play a major role in killing flukes and nematodes that have IgG or complement bound to their surface.
    D. Eosinophils have limited phagocytic and bactericidal activity and may play a role in destroying neoplastic cells.
    E. Eosinophils have long circulating half-lives.

18. Causes of peripheral eosinophilia may include all of the following except:
    A. Allergic skin disease
    B. Heartworm disease
    C. Whipworm infection
    D. Mast cell tumors
    E. Hypereosinophilic syndrome

19. Specific macrophage functions include:
    A. Phagocytosis
    B. Regulation of the inflammatory response via release of inflammatory mediators
    C. Antigen-processing for presentation to lymphocytes
    D. Regulation of body iron stores
    E. All of the above

20. Monocytosis can indicate:
    A. The presence of inflammation
    B. Demand for phagocytosis
    C. Tissue necrosis
    D. A "stress response" induced by high circulating glucocorticoids
    E. All of the above

21. Which of the following is correct?
    A. Monocytes originate in extramedullary sites.
    B. Monocytes are released into the peripheral blood as immature cells.
    C. Monocytes have a large bone marrow storage pool.
    D. Monocytes recirculate and have bi-directional movement.
    E. Monocytosis occurs with chronic inflammation only.

22. Peripheral lymphocytes:
    A. Are capable of phagocytosis.
    B. Are approximately 70% bone marrow derived (B lymphocytes) and approximately 30% thymus derived (T-lymphocytes).
    C. Have the unique ability to recirculate.
    D. Survive in the body for only a total of 6-14 hours.
    E. All of the above are correct.

23. Causes of severe lymphopenia (<700 lymphocytes/ul) include all of the following except:
    A. Epinephrine release
    B. Lymphangectasia
    C. Lymphosarcoma
    D. Chylothorax
    E. Thoracic duct obstruction

24. Lymphocytosis in dogs may be caused by all of the following except:
    A. Excitement
    B. Recent vaccination
    C. Inflammatory conditions associated with antigenic stimulation.
    D. Lymphosarcoma
    E. Lymphocytic leukemia

25. A canine patient is suspected of ingesting a coumarin-based rodenticide. Of the following tests, which should show evidence of abnormality first?
    A. Prothrombin Time (PT)
    B. Activated Partial Thromboplastin Time (APTT)
    C. Activated Coagulation Time (ACT)
    D. Thrombin Time (TT)
    E. Fibrinogen concentration

26. The most appropriate test to determine hemorrhagic potential in a patient with known von Willebrand's factor (vWf) deficiency is
    A. The platelet count.
    B. von Willebrand factor (vWf) quantitation.
    C. The buccal mucosal bleeding time (BMBT).
    D. Factor VIII (FVIII) quantitation.
    E. The Activated Coagulation Time (ACT) test.

27. A canine patient has a prolonged buccal mucosal bleeding time (BMBT), appropriate platelet numbers and appropriate PT and APTT tests. This suggests
    A. An endothelial cell or platelet functional problem.
    B. A coagulation factor deficiency, probably in the intrinsic path.
    C. A coagulation factor deficiency, probably in the extrinsic path.
    D. A coagulation factor deficiency involving the common path.
    E. Excessive fibrinolysis.

28. An elderly male dog has clinical evidence of hemorrhagic diatheses following splenectomy for hemangiosarcoma. The platelet count is moderately reduced; fibrinogen concentration is also reduced. APTT is prolonged. Fibrin degradation products (FDPs) are increased. This constellation of laboratory test results suggests:
    A. The neoplasm has metastasized.
    B. This patient has thrombus formation.
    C. DIC.
    D. This patient has an additional problem, probably vitamin K inhibition.
    E. Factor VII deficiency.

29. Which of the following are consistent with inflammatory leukograms?
    A. Persistent eosinophilia,
    B. Monocytosis
    C. Neutrophilic left shift
    D. Absolute neutrophilias of greater than 25,000/μl
    E. All of the above

30. Which characteristic of stress leukograms is most consistent?
    A. Lymphocyte counts between 750/μl and 1500/μl
    B. Eosinopenia
    C. Marked neutrophilia
    D. Moderate monocytosis
    E. Nonregenerative anemia

# 14

# Appendix

## Self-Test Answers

# ANSWERS

1. Which of the following is incorrect?

   **B. Erythropoietin stimulates white blood cell (WBC) production**

2. Which of the following is/are correct?

   **E. All of the above**

3. Which of the following is incorrect?

   **D. Feline hemoglobin is less susceptible to oxidation than canine hemoglobin**

4. The proper term for poikilocytes with 2-10 blunt elongate finger-like surface projections is:

   **A. Acanthocytes**

5. Which of the following is/are correct?

   **C. Crenation is more prominent in films made from EDTA-antico agulated blood than in films made from fresh non-anticoagulated blood.**

6. Regenerative anemias:

   **E. All of the above**

7. Which type of anemia best fits a reticulocyte count of 100,000 reticulocytes/ul and a decreased total plasma protein?

   **A. Blood loss anemias**

8. Conditions which can cause immune-mediated hemolytic disease include:

   **E. All of the above**

9. Which of the following is correct?

   **A. Maturation defect anemias have nonregenerative peripheral blood patterns but erythroid hyperplasia in the bone marrow.**

10. Which of the following is/are incorrect about polycythemia?

    **E. is most commonly caused by polycythemia vera**

11. Laboratory features of relative polycythemia may include:

    **E. All of the above**

12. Which of the following is correct?
    **E. All of the above**

13. Which of the following can affect the neutrophil count in peripheral blood?
    **E. All of the above**

14. Mechanisms of neutropenia include:
    **E. All of the above**

15. Causes of neutrophilia include all of the following except:
    **E. Endotoxemia**

16. Which of the following best describes a leukogram characterized by a mild leukocytosis with mature neutrophilia, lymphopenia, eosinopenia, and mild monocytosis?
    **A. Stress leukogram**

17. Which of the following are incorrect about eosinophils?
    **E. Eosinophils have long circulating half-lives.**

18. Causes of peripheral eosinophilia may include all of the following except:
    **C. Whipworm infection**

19. Specific macrophage functions include:
    **E. All of the above**

20. Monocytosis can indicate:
    **E. All of the above**

21. Which of the following is correct?
    **B. Monocytes are released into the peripheral blood as immature cells.**

22. Peripheral lymphocytes:
    **C. Have the unique ability to recirculate**

23. Causes of severe lymphopenia (<700 lymphocytes/ul) include all of the following except:
    **A. Epinephrine release**

24. Lymphocytosis in dogs may be caused by all of the following except:
    **A. Excitement**

25. A canine patient is suspected of ingesting a coumarin-based rodenticide. Of the following tests, which should show evidence of abnormality first?
    **A. Prothrombin Time (PT)**

26. The most appropriate test to determine hemorrhagic potential in a patient with known von Willebrand's factor (vWf) deficiency is
    **C. The buccal mucosal bleeding time (BMBT).**

27. A canine patient has a prolonged buccal mucosal bleeding time (BMBT), appropriate platelet numbers, and appropriate PT and APTT tests. This suggests
    **A. An endothelial cell or platelet functional problem.**

28. An elderly male dog has clinical evidence of hemorrhagic diatheses following splenectomy for hemangiosarcoma. The platelet count is moderately reduced, fibrinogen concentration is also reduced. APTT is prolonged.  Fibrin degradation products (FDPs) are increased. This constellation of laboratory test results suggests
    **C. DIC.**

29. Which of the following are consistent with inflammatory leukograms?
    **E. All of the above**

30. Which characteristic of stress leukograms is most consistent:?
    **A.  Lymphocyte counts between 750/$\mu$l and 1500/$\mu$l**

# INDEX

Griseofulvin, 73

# H

*Haemobartonella*
  *canis*, 53
    anemia due to, 227–228
  *felis*, 50, 51f, 52f, 209–210
    organisms of, 40
Haemobartonellosis
  canine, 53
  feline, 50–52, 209–210
Halothane, 133t
Heart defect, 215–216
Heart disease, mechanical hemolysis
  with, 56
Heartworm disease, 56
Heinz bodies
  in canine blood, 50f, 51f
  in false elevated WBC counts, 24
  in feline blood, 38f, 201f
  formation of, 31, 48
  hemolysis of in cats, 50
  methylene blue staining of, 13
  oxidized hemoglobin and, 48–49
  in poikilocytosis, 36
Heinz body anemia
  blood films in, 50
  diagnosis of, 50
  eccentrocytes in, 49
  oxidizing substances in, 49
  pathogenesis of, 48
Heinz body hemolytic anemia
  drug-induced, 199–200, 201f
  in feline blood, 37f
Hemangiosarcoma
  in mechanical hemolysis, 56
  ruptured splenic, 219–220, 221f
Hemantinics, 219
Hematocrit methods, 16–17
Hematology
  communicating need for, 7–8
  communicating results of, 8
  in-clinic versus outside laboratory, 6–7
  indications for, 5–6
  laboratory costs in, 8
  laboratory methods in, 10–28
Hematopoiesis, cyclic, 79
Hemoconcentration, 18
Hemocytometer, 19
  grid lines of, 20f
  in platelet count, 21
Hemoglobin
  concentration of, 18–19
  Heinz bodies and, 199
  oxidation of, 31
    in cats, 50
    in cats versus dogs, 238, 246
  oxidized, 48–49
Hemoglobinemia, 140
  in intravascular hemolysis, 45
Hemoglobinometers, 18

Hemoglobinuria, 140
  in regenerative hemolytic anemia, 45
Hemograms
  interpretation of, 136–144
  platelet, 143–144
  red cell, 139–142
  white cell, 136–139
Hemolysis
  diagnosis of, 140–141
  mechanical, 56
  with pyruvate kinase deficiency, 55
Hemolytic anemia
  causes of, 199, 209
  drug-induced Heinz body, 199–200,
    201f
  immune-mediated, 45–48
    conditions causing, 239, 246
  neutrophilia and, 79
  regenerative, 45–52
Hemolytic disease, 54–56
  abnormal red cells in, 140–141
  in canine blood, 38–39f
  immune-mediated canine, 171–172,
    173f
Hemolytic uremic syndrome, 126
Hemorrhage
  in canine bone marrow, 60f
  generalized systemic, 119
  in reactive thrombocytosis, 129
Hemorrhagic anemia, 44
  neutrophilia and, 79
Hemorrhagic diatheses, 243, 248
Hemostasis, 113
Heparin
  in blood collection, 11
  inhibiting coagulation, 94
  modifying platelet function, 133*t*
  in thrombocytopenia, 128
*Hepatozoon*, 82
Hetastarch, 133*t*
Hexose monophosphate shunt, 31
Histamine
  basophil release of, 94
  release of, 88
*Histoplasma*
  in neutrophil cytoplasm, 82
  phagocytized, 103f
Histoplasmosis, 101
Hocytes, 108
Hookworm disease
  in *Babesia canis*, 168, 169f
  ova of, 167
Hormone treatment, 132
Howell-Jolly bodies
  in canine blood, 33f
  in canine red cells, 31
  in feline blood, 34f
Humoral immunity, 105
Hyperadrenocorticism, 149
  in prothrombotic states, 132
Hypereosinophilic syndrome, 89
Hyperglobulinemia, 77

# L

# M

RBCs. *See* Red blood cells
Red blood cell counts, 140–141
  algorithms for, 25–26
  with impedance counter, 22
  overestimates of, 23
Red blood cell precursors, selective
    destruction of, 62
Red blood cells
  abnormalities of, 5
  abnormally shaped, 36–39
  agglutination of, 172f
    in IMHA, 45, 46f
  aggregation of, 14
  artifacts in, 40–43
  circulation of, 238, 246
  crenated with rouleaux formation, 185f
  destruction of, 30
  differentiation of, 22
  function of, 30–31
  with Heinz bodies, 24
  hemogram interpretation of, 139–142
  hypochromic, 165f
  in immune-mediate hemolytic disease,
    172f
  immune-mediated destruction of, 209
  increased circulating mass of, 64
  lysing of, 24
  manual counting of, 19
  morphology of, 141
    assessment of, 16
    in disease, 35–39
    normal canine, 31–33
    normal feline, 34
    normal, 117f
  overstaining of, 14f, 41
  parasites and inclusions of, 28
  phagocytized, 238, 246
  physiology of, 31
  polychromatic, 24
  polychromatophilic, 163–164
  production of, 30
    ineffective, 57
  quantitative data on, 139–140
  quantity of
    in anemia, 44–64
    in polycythemia, 64–67
  susceptibility to lysis, 10
Refractometers, hand held, 18f
Refractory bubbles
  in feline blood, 41f
  on red cell surface, 40
Regenerative anemia, 44
  blood loss/hemorrhage in, 44
  hemolytic, 45–52
Reiderform, 108
Renal disease anemia, 62f
Reticulated platelet count, 114
Reticulocyte counts
  in blood loss anemia, 239, 246
  manual, 19
  methylene blue in, 13
  in regenerative anemia, 44
Reticulocytes

aggregate and punctate, 38f
  in canine blood, 33f
  in feline blood, 201f
Reticulocytosis, 168
Rodenticide, tests for, 242, 248
Romanowsky stains, 13
  for feline platelet morphology, 116
  for platelet morphology, 115
  stain precipitate on, 40
Rouleaux formation
  versus autoagglutination, 48
  in canine red cells, 31, 32f
  crenated RBCs with, 185f
  in feline blood, 34f
  scanning for, 14

# S

Schistocytes
  in canine blood, 39f
  in poikilocytosis, 36
  in thrombosis and DIC, 221f
Self-drawing evacuated tubes, 11
Self-test
  answers, 246–248
  questions, 238–243
Semi-automated cell counters, 22
Serology, 125
Sertoli cell tumor, 179–180
Serum albumin, 18
Serum protein, 18
Sickness, defined, 5
Smears. *See* Blood smears
Snake envenomation, 235
Sodium citrate, 10
Spherocytes
  in immune-mediated hemolytic
    anemia, 46, 173f
  in poikilocytosis, 36
  regenerative anemia with, 37f
Spherocytosis
  in canine blood, 47f
  in feline blood, 47f
Spheroenchinocytes
  in canine blood, 221f
  in pyruvate kinase deficiency, 55
Spitz thrombopathia, 134
Splenectomy, 129
Splenic pool, platelets in, 113–114
Springer Spaniels, phosphofructokinase
    deficiency in, 56
Stain precipitate, 13
  in canine blood, 42f
  in feline blood, 42f
  of red blood cells, 40–41
Staining, 13
  common artifacts and issues of, 13
Stem cell differentiation, 70
Stomatocytes, 36
Stress, hemogram evidence of, 136
Stress-induced neutrophilia, 76